W9-BCE-984

Second Edition

Study Guide for

*F*undamentals

of Nursing

Caring and Clinical Judgment

Mary Ann Hogan, MSN, RN, CS
Clinical Assistant Professor
University of Massachusetts Amherst
Amherst, Massachusetts

Marshelle Thobaben, MS, RN, PHN, APNP, FNP
Professor and Community Health and Psychiatric Nursing Consultant
Department of Nursing
Humboldt State University
Arcata, California

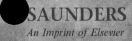

SAUNDERS
An Imprint of Elsevier

SAUNDERS
An Imprint of Elsevier

11830 Westline Industrial Drive
St. Louis, Missouri 63146

STUDY GUIDE FOR FUNDAMENTALS OF NURSING:
CARING AND CLINICAL JUDGMENT
Copyright © 2004, Elsevier (USA). All rights reserved.

No part of this publication may be reproduced or transmitted in any form or by any means, electronic or mechanical, including photocopying, recording, or any information storage and retrieval system, without permission in writing from the publisher. Permissions may be sought directly from Elsevier's Health Sciences Rights Department in Philadelphia, PA, USA: phone: (+1) 215 238 7869, fax: (+1) 215 238 2239, e-mail: healthpermissions@elsevier.com. You may also complete your request on-line via the Elsevier Science homepage (http://www.elsevier.com), by selecting 'Customer Support' and then 'Obtaining Permissions'.

Notice

Nursing is an ever-changing field. Standard safety precautions must be followed, but as new research and clinical experience broaden our knowledge, changes in treatment and drug therapy become necessary or appropriate. Readers are advised to check the product information currently provided by the manufacturer of each drug to be administered to verify the recommended dose, the method and duration of administration, and the contraindications. It is the responsibility of the licensed health care provider, relying on experience and knowledge of the patient, to determine dosages and the best treatment for the patient. Neither the publisher nor the editor assumes any responsibility for any injury and/or damage to persons or property.

The Publisher

Previous edition copyrighted 2000

ISBN-13: 978-0-7216-0098-7
ISBN-10: 0-7216-0098-0

Executive Vice President, Nursing & Health Professions: Sally Schrefer
Executive Editor: Susan Epstein
Developmental Editor: Linda Stagg
Publishing Services Manager: Gayle May
Production Manager: Joseph Selby
Designer: Kathi Gosche

Printed in the United States

Last digit is the print number: 9   8   7   6   5   4   3

Preface

The *Study Guide* for Harkreader and Hogan's *Fundamentals of Nursing: Caring and Clinical Judgment* was developed to assist you, the nursing student, to understand and apply important concepts presented in the textbook. As a beginning nursing student, you will probably be expected to learn a tremendous amount of material in a relatively short time. The *Study Guide* was written to help you make good use of your valuable study time.

Each *Study Guide* chapter follows a specific format:

- **Purpose:** Each chapter begins with a brief purpose statement that summarizes in a few sentences the content of the corresponding textbook chapter.
- **Learning Objectives:** The learning objectives from the textbook are reproduced to help you focus on the critical elements of each chapter as you study.
- **Matching:** Matching exercises allow you to test your recall of basic terminology from each chapter.
- **True or False:** True or false exercises allow you to test your understanding of factual information presented in the text of the chapter. The answer key at the end of the book corrects the false statements.
- **Fill-in-the-Blanks:** Fill-in-the-blanks exercises help you master comprehension of important fundamental concepts and apply them in a specific context.
- **Exercising Your Clinical Judgment:** "Exercising Your Clinical Judgment" sections use a case study (often the familiar one presented in the textbook chapter) and NCLEX-style multiple-choice questions to give you practice in applying clinical reasoning skills.
- **Test Yourself:** The "Test Yourself" sections present a series of freestanding NCLEX-style multiple-choice questions to give you practice in test-taking and help you prepare for exams.

The answers to all of the exercises are provided at the end of the book for immediate feedback on the degree to which you have mastered the chapter contents.

Following the answer section, you'll find **Performance Checklists** that correspond to the Procedures in the textbook. Each one presents the essential elements of the corresponding Procedure. The checklists are designed for use in two ways. First, you may use them for individual review as you practice performing Procedures. Second, an instructor may use them to test your mastery of the Procedures. The format allows the instructor not only to rate your performance, but also to provide specific comments that will enhance your learning and help you to refine your skills.

We hope you find the *Study Guide* to be not only useful but also enjoyable for study. We also wish you success as you begin your career, and we hope that you will quickly discover all the richness, fulfillment, and satisfaction that nursing has to offer!

Mary Ann Hogan, MSN, RN, CS
Marshelle Thobaben, MS, RN, PHN, APNP, FNP

Contents

The Nursing Profession

PURPOSE

This chapter provides a broad overview of the nursing profession. It describes significant events in history and how they have affected the evolution of the nursing profession. The chapter also examines the various roles you will have as a nurse, professional nursing practice standards, advanced education options, and current issues of concern to those in the nursing profession.

MATCHING

1. ____ client advocate

2. ____ continuing education

3. ____ in-service programs

4. ____ nursing

5. ____ professionalism

6. ____ registered nurse (RN)

7. ____ standards of nursing practice

    a. an accountable discipline guided by science, theory, a code of ethics, and the art of care and comfort to treat human responses to health and illness

    b. the nurse who assists clients in expressing their rights whenever necessary

    c. behavior that upholds the status, methods, character, and standards of a given profession

    d. informal courses that assist professional nurses in developing and maintaining clinical expertise and knowledge that promotes the quality of nursing care

    e. a set of nursing actions that are generally agreed upon by nurses as constituting safe and effective client care

    f. a nurse who is registered to practice nursing in a particular state after graduating from a state-approved educational program and passing the National Council Licensing Examination for Registered Nurses

    g. programs designed to increase knowledge and skills needed for nursing practice in a particular agency; topics often relate to new policies, procedures, or equipment

TRUE OR FALSE

8. ____ Nursing has been defined in many different ways, but the caregiving focus has remained humanistic and holistic.

9. ____ Nursing as a profession is under the domain of medicine and is regulated by medicine.

10. ____ The American Nurses Association is the representative professional association for nurses in the United States.

11. ____ Florence Nightingale is considered by many to be the founder of nursing.

12. ____ Isabel Hampton Robb founded the organization that later became the American Nurses Association.

13. ____ A doctoral degree program is considered entry level education in nursing.

14. ____ A nurse who is planning the best method of care delivery for a client is engaged in the nursing role of rehabilitator.

15. ____ Specialty nursing organizations often offer certification for nurses practicing in that specialty.

16. ____ There continues to be a steady increase in the number of registered nurses employed in ambulatory care and community settings.

17. ____ The nursing profession has consistently tried to be removed from the political arena.

FILL-IN-THE-BLANKS

18. During the _____ _____, the bubonic plague contributed to the founding of many nursing orders, including the Augustinian sisters.

Copyright © 2004, Elsevier Science (USA). All Rights Reserved.

19. The book Notes on Nursing: What It Is and What It Is Not was written by _____ _____.

20. The value of primary prevention became understood in America during the American _____ War.

21. The first nurse to be appointed a university professorship at Columbia University Teachers College was _____ _____ _____.

22. In 1893, Lillian Wald founded _____ _____.nursing when she opened the Henry Street Settlement Service in New York City.

23. *Nursing's Agenda for Health Care Reform* focuses on _____ _____, _____, and _____ _____ .

24. A nurse practitioner, nurse educator, or nurse administrator often completes a 2-year _____ _____ program.

25. Continuing education is mandatory in some states to maintain _____ _____ .

26. A Nurse Practice Act defines the scope of nursing practice in a _____ .

EXERCISING YOUR CLINICAL JUDGMENT

Kate Lorraine is a 22-year-old nursing graduate. She has just taken her first job in a subacute unit of a local rehabilitation nursing center. Kate is highly motivated to grow in her professional practice, and to deliver quality nursing care to her clients.

27. To be aware of her specific legal responsibilities in her daily nursing practice, Kate should become familiar with which of the following?
    1. State Nurse Practice Act
    2. National League for Nursing (NLN) accreditation criteria
    3. Association of Rehabilitation Nurses (ARN) guidelines
    4. American Nurses' Association (ANA) standards of nursing practice

28. As Kate is working on the evening shift, she observes one client looking through the bedside table drawer of another client. Kate intervenes, knowing which of the following nursing roles assumes the highest priority at this moment?
    1. Caregiver
    2. Communicator
    3. Client advocate
    4. Manager

29. Kate takes a supper break with a nursing colleague. They talk about some of the flyers for continuing education programs that are hanging on the break room bulletin board. Kate begins to think about the importance of acquiring continuing education units (CEUs) to maintain which of the following?
    1. Opportunities for future pay increases
    2. Professional licensure
    3. Status among her colleagues
    4. Membership in the American Nurses Association (ANA)

30. Kate overhears that another nurse has just received generalist certification from the American Nurses Credentialing Center (ANCC). She is aware that this nurse has which of the following as a minimum educational degree?
    1. Associate's degree
    2. Bachelor's degree
    3. Master's degree
    4. Doctorate degree

TEST YOURSELF

31. Nursing can best be defined as a discipline that focuses on which of the following items?
    1. Human responses to health and illness
    2. A wide variety of disease states
    3. The interaction between nurses and other disciplines
    4. The women's movement in the United States

32. The nurse's role as a case manager, who reviews and coordinates care in various health settings, developed as a result of which of the following recent trends in health care?
    1. Increased technology
    2. Concern for quality regardless of cost
    3. Managed care
    4. Computerization

33. Which of the following is the official publication by the American Nurses Association for registered nurses?
    1. *RN*
    2. *American Journal of Nursing*
    3. *Nursing*
    4. *Nursing Research*

34. With the changing health care delivery system, which of the following most common settings for nursing practice is experiencing a decline in numbers of employed nurses?
    1. Rehabilitation centers
    2. Home care
    3. Ambulatory care centers
    4. Hospitals

Copyright © 2004, Elsevier Science (USA). All Rights Reserved.

35. Experts predict that in the future which of the
following is most likely to take place in the health
care arena and affect the practice of nursing?
    1. Nurses will work in 24-hour physician-managed
       clinics.
    2. Hospital stays will become longer once again.
    3. The focus of nursing will revert back to illness
       rather than health.
    4. Nurse practitioners will provide services
       traditionally provided by physicians.

Copyright © 2004, Elsevier Science (USA). All Rights Reserved.

Legal and Ethical Context of Practice

2

PURPOSE

This chapter discusses the legal foundation for your nursing practice, and explores the theories and principles of ethics. It provides information about the legal and professional regulation of nursing practice, client rights, quality of care improvement initiatives, and methods to safeguard your nursing practice against legal threats. It also provides guidelines for ethical decision making that can be applied systematically to nursing practice.

MATCHING

1. ____ accreditation
2. ____ advance directive
3. ____ assault
4. ____ autonomy
5. ____ battery
6. ____ beneficence
7. ____ certification
8. ____ civil law
9. ____ common law
10. ____ confidentiality
11. ____ contract
12. ____ credentialing
13. ____ criminal law
14. ____ defamation
15. ____ defendant
16. ____ durable power of attorney for health care
17. ____ ethics

18. ____ false imprisonment
19. ____ fraud
20. ____ informed consent
21. ____ invasion of privacy
22. ____ law
23. ____ liability
24. ____ license
25. ____ living will
26. ____ malpractice
27. ____ morals
28. ____ negligence
29. ____ nonmaleficence
30. ____ plaintiff
31. ____ procedural law
32. ____ professional misconduct
33. ____ registration
34. ____ statutory law
35. ____ tort
36. ____ values
37. ____ values clarification
38. ____ veracity

a. includes standards and rules applicable to our interactions with one another that are recognized, affirmed, and enforced through judicial decisions

b. the individual against whom a lawsuit is filed

c. involves the legal right of a client to receive adequate and accurate information about medical condition and treatment

4 Copyright © 2004, Elsevier Science (USA). All Rights Reserved.

d. acts of negligence by a professional person as compared with the actions of another professional person in similar circumstances

e. violations of a Nurse Practice Act that can result in disciplinary action against a nurse

f. the client's right to privacy in the health care delivery system

g. a process that monitors an educational program's ability to meet predetermined standards for students' outcomes

h. can occur when the nurse unreasonably intrudes upon the client's private affairs

i. occurs when harm or injury is caused by an act of either omission or commission by a layperson

j. adhering to the truth

k. law enacted by the state or federal legislative branch of government

l. any legal written document that provides direction for health care for a future time when the person is unable to make treatment choices; may be a living will or durable power of attorney for health care

m. an agreement between two or more individuals that creates certain rights and obligations in exchange for goods or services

n. a body of rules of action or conduct prescribed by a "controlling authority"

o. the party bringing a lawsuit who alleges certain facts and outcomes

p. a process by an applicant provides specific information to the state agency administering the nursing registration process

q. an attempt or threat to touch another person unjustly

r. the methods by which the nursing profession attempts to ensure and maintain the competency of its practitioners

s. standards of conduct that represent the ideal in human behavior to which society expects its members to adhere

t. a document that designates a person to make decisions about the client's medical treatment in the event that the client becomes unable to do so

u. involves the restraining, with or without force, against that person's wishes

v. a civil wrong by one person against another person or his or her property

w. the actual willful touching of another person that may or may not cause harm

x. defines specific behaviors determined to be inappropriate in the orderly functioning of society

y. establishes the manner of proceeding used to enforce a specific legal right or obtain redress

z. implies a legal obligation for which the nurse can be held responsible and accountable

aa. a voluntary process by which a nurse can be granted recognition for meeting certain criteria established by a nongovernmental association

bb. either a false communication or a careless disregard for the truth that results in damage to one's reputation; can take two forms—libel and slander

cc. grants the owner formal permission from a constituted authority to practice a particular profession

dd. the false representation of some fact with the intention that it will be acted upon by another person

ee. regulates disputes between individuals and/or individuals and groups

ff. refers to a person's right to make individual choices; to self-determine

gg. ideals, beliefs, and patterns of behavior that are prized and chosen by a person, group, or society

hh. the branch of philosophy that attempts to determine what constitutes good, bad, right, and wrong in human behavior

ii. the promotion of good

jj. an advanced directive in which a person provides written instructions about his/her wishes for the use of life-sustaining measures or other treatment options to help in decision making at a time when that person is unable to make decisions for himself

kk. requires the practitioner to do no harm

ll. allows you to identify your personal values and develop self-awareness

TRUE OR FALSE

39. ____ A nurse overheard making vicious untrue comments about a coworker could be charged with defamation.

40. ____ False imprisonment does not include refusing to let clients leave the hospital against their wishes, as long as it is in their best interests to stay.

Copyright © 2004, Elsevier Science (USA). All Rights Reserved.

41. ____ A person who has been declared incompetent by the court is considered to lack the capacity for entering into a contract.

42. ____ A nurse who diverts and sells narcotics can be tried in the court system under civil law.

43. ____ Failing to practice within legal boundaries of nursing practice could result in professional discipline, civil or criminal lawsuits, or employer disciplinary action.

44. ____ The American Nurses' Association is the body that has the power to change a Nurse Practice Act.

45. ____ A nursing school that is accredited meets predetermined standards for student outcomes.

46. ____ The process of registration or the renewal of registration helps to ensure that a state has the most current information about a person granted a nursing license.

47. ____ Values shape decisions in everyday life, from the clothes we wear to movies we prefer.

48. ____ Maintaining client confidentiality means not discussing client issues in hallways, elevators, hospital parking lots, or at home with family and friends.

49. ____ An example of applying the principle of veracity is not telling a terminally ill client his or her prognosis.

50. ____ When two or more principles are in conflict or when choices are favorable, you have an ethical dilemma.

51. ____ In the United States, the American Nurses' Association Code for Nurses is the document governing ethical nursing practice.

52. ____ A common ethical problem you may encounter is unit staffing patterns that negatively influence the provision of safe nursing care.

FILL-IN-THE-BLANKS

53. A nurse who administers an injection to a client despite the client's refusal has committed _____ .

54. A nurse who is threatened with loss of license is given the right to a fair hearing under _____ law.

55. A nurse who sits for an examination administered by a specialty nursing organization is seeking _____ .

56. The process whereby a union negotiates with an employer for nurses' salaries is termed _____ _____ .

57. Before undergoing any invasive procedure, the client must give_____ _____ .

58. By avoiding conversations about clients in elevators and hallways, a nurse is protecting the client's right to _____ .

59. A nurse would fill out an _____ _____ if a client slipped and fell on a wet floor on the nursing unit.

60. The study of _____ entails the examination of human behavior in terms of what ought to be done in the course of human interactions, and it seeks to provide guidelines or principles as a way to direct human interaction.

61. Values are learned behaviors that are influenced by _____, ethnicity, education, and _____ _____ .

62. Confidentiality means maintaining another's _____ by safeguarding information that is entrusted to you.

63. _____ is the complement of beneficence.

64. Durable powers of attorney for health care and living wills are both included in the client's _____ record.

EXERCISING YOUR CLINICAL JUDGMENT

The registered nurse has arrived on the clinical unit in the hospital to begin the shift. The nurse will be assigned to a group of seven clients, and has been designated as the charge nurse for the day as well.

65. While beginning to listen to intershift report at the nurses' station, a nurse notes that a client is within earshot. The client states that he would like a cup of coffee until the meal trays arrive. The most appropriate action by the nurse would be to:
    1. ask the client to wait until after report.
    2. tell the client that coffee is unavailable at this time.
    3. ask a nursing assistant to bring coffee to the desk for the client, and continue with report.
    4. ask someone to bring coffee to the client's room, and continue with report after the client leaves.

Copyright © 2004, Elsevier Science (USA). All Rights Reserved.

66. A nurse receives a telephone call stating that a client will be admitted with suspected tuberculosis in the infectious stage. The nurse would plan care for this client using infection control guidelines from the:
    1. Centers for Disease Control and Prevention.
    2. Occupational Safety and Health Administration.
    3. state Nurse Practice Act.
    4. American Nurses' Association.

67. A nurse is documenting care given to an assigned client. The nurse would do which of the following to make an appropriate legal entry in the client's medical record?
    1. Use descriptive words such as "good" or "angry."
    2. Record measurable and factual information about the client's condition.
    3. Use correcting fluid after making a mistake.
    4. Sign each entry using initials and license number.

TEST YOURSELF

68. You and your classmate discuss your clients in the parking lot. You think that others are not listening to your conversation. Which of the following principles did you breach?
    1. Autonomy
    2. Fidelity
    3. Confidentiality
    4. Beneficence

69. You tell your client that you will give her pain medication at 10 AM. You follow through and give the medication when you stated. You are supporting which ethical principle when you follow through on your commitment?
    1. Autonomy
    2. Beneficence
    3. Nonmaleficence
    4. Fidelity

70. Your client, who has a terminal illness and is expected to live for 6 months, is alert, oriented, and competent. She has very definite wishes about when life-sustaining treatment should be terminated. To support the client's self-determination, the best advice to give her is to:
    1. tell her primary care provider about her wishes.
    2. have a living will.
    3. have a durable power of attorney.
    4. talk with the institution's ethics committee.

71. A nurse is being charged with malpractice. The element of malpractice that is proven by determining that the nurse did not meet the standard of care is:
    1. duty.
    2. breach of duty.
    3. causation.
    4. damages.

72. A nurse is admitting a client who wishes to have "do not resuscitate" status. The nurse determines whether the client has a copy of which of the following items to add to the client's record?
    1. Letter of intent
    2. Physician letter of approval
    3. Advance directive
    4. Last will and testament

73. A nurse is uncertain whether the client understood information about an upcoming invasive diagnostic procedure as presented by a physician. Which of the following factors may invalidate this client's consent?
    1. Emotional status only
    2. Intelligence
    3. Educational level
    4. Emotional or physical barriers

74. A nurse who works with a client population with a high incidence of hypertension (high blood pressure) attends a full-day workshop providing information on nursing management of this disorder. This nurse is striving to maintain which of the following types of competency in nursing practice?
    1. Technical
    2. Cognitive
    3. Interpersonal
    4. Global

75. Three components of a moral conflict include:
    1. personal values, uncertainty, and distress.
    2. choosing, prizing, and acting.
    3. uncertainty, dilemma, and distress.
    4. identifying, examining, and evaluating solutions.

76. You answer a client's questions about his or her diabetes, even though it would have been more comfortable for you to tell the client "not to worry" about the disorder. Which ethical principle applies in this situation?
    1. Autonomy
    2. Virtue
    3. Veracity
    4. Beneficence

Copyright © 2004, Elsevier Science (USA). All Rights Reserved.

77. Using the six-step ethical decision-making process, step 2 is gathering pertinent data. Which of the following questions should you ask to attempt to gather data about an ethical dilemma?
    1. Do institutional values and systems support the nursing decisions made?
    2. With whom must the final decision be made, and is that person competent or empowered to make decisions?
    3. Is the situation truly an ethical dilemma?
    4. What is the effect on those involved?

78. The American Hospital Association's Patient's Bill of Rights supports the client's right to refuse a recommended treatment or plan of care to the extent permitted by law and hospital policy. Which ethical principle does the bill of rights support?
    1. Nonmaleficence
    2. Autonomy
    3. Beneficence
    4. Veracity

Copyright © 2004, Elsevier Science (USA). All Rights Reserved.

Cultural Context of Practice

PURPOSE

This chapter discusses concepts of culture and ethnicity as they relate to nursing care. It provides an overview of transcultural nursing and gives suggestions for performing a transcultural assessment. It also explores basic aspects of selected cultures and their effect on the successful delivery of nursing care.

MATCHING

1. ____ cultural competence
2. ____ culture
3. ____ diversity
4. ____ ethnic
5. ____ ethnicity
6. ____ ethnocentrism
7. ____ humanistic care
8. ____ multicultural society
9. ____ stereotyping
10. ____ transcultural nursing
11. ____ universality

a. groups of people of the same race or national origin within a larger cultural system who are distinctive based on traditions of religion, language, or appearance

b. culturally competent nursing care focused on differences and similarities among cultures, with respect to caring, health, and illness, based on the client's cultural values, beliefs, and practices

c. a society composed of more than one culture or subculture

d. the assumption that an attribute present in some members of a group is present in all members of a group

e. having enough knowledge of cultural groups that are different from your own to be able to interact with a member of a group in a manner that makes the person feel respected and understood

f. reflects the characteristics a group may share in some combination

g. a common mode or value of caring or a prevailing pattern of care across cultures

h. the belief that one's own ethnic beliefs, customs, and attitudes are the correct and thus superior ones

i. a patterned behavioral response that develops over time as a consequence of imprinting the mind through social and religious structures and intellectual and artistic manifestations

j. the differences in modes or patterns of care between cultures, including specific patterns of care within cultural groups

k. includes understanding and knowing a client in as natural or human a way as possible while helping or guiding the client to achieve certain goals, make improvements, reduce discomfort, or face disability or death

TRUE OR FALSE

12. ____ One benefit of providing care within the framework of the client's culture is that it can improve compliance with the health regimen.

13. ____ The majority of Asian-Americans would prefer acupuncture to Western approaches to analgesia.

14. ____ The nurse who wishes to provide culturally competent care must have a willingness to compromise with the client about some aspects of care.

15. ____ The cultural phenomenon of space in the transcultural assessment model refers to personal space.

Copyright © 2004, Elsevier Science (USA). All Rights Reserved.

16. ____ A person who is future-oriented in terms of time often has difficulty accepting a plan of care that conflicts with traditional treatments.

17. ____ When communicating with a client from another culture, it is helpful to use eye contact, touch, and seating arrangements that are comfortable for that client.

18. ____ The African-American culture as a group values religion and the power of prayer.

19. ____ Mexican-Americans are more likely to perceive life as being under the influence of a divine will.

20. ____ Husbands and elders have authority over wives and children in the family/social structure of the Chinese-American culture.

21. ____ Native Americans subscribe to the germ theory of medicine.

FILL-IN-THE-BLANKS

22. A nurse who helps a client to continue an important cultural practice during illness is engaged in cultural care _____ or _____.

23. A nurse who changes personal behavior or actions to be more fully understood or accepted by the client is engaged in cultural care _____ or _____.

24. _____ is the attribute of cultural competency in which the health care provider recognizes the values and beliefs of both the client and self.

25. _____ _____ is the element of transcultural assessment that indicates clients' beliefs about their ability to control disease.

26. The _____ -American cultural group has readily assimilated into the cultural mainstream of U.S. society.

27. Sickle cell disease is a genetic disorder that is prevalent in the _____-American population.

28. _____ -Americans are the fastest growing minority group in the United States.

29. The cultural group that adjusts personal diet to meet the yin-yang quality of a disease is the _____ -American group.

30. Type 2 diabetes mellitus has high prevalence and tends to occur in the teens and twenties among the _____ _____.

31. In traditional Navajo culture, health reflects living in total _____ with nature and having the ability to survive under extremely difficult circumstances.

EXERCISING YOUR CLINICAL JUDGMENT

Mrs. Haygood is a 50-year-old African-American client who has been hospitalized for cardiovascular surgery. She has three grown children and works part time as a receptionist for a local business. A nurse has been assigned as the primary nurse for this client during her postoperative course of recovery.

32. A certified nursing assistant (CNA) tells the nurse that the client speaks "black English" when conversing with family and friends, and reverts to standard English when speaking with nursing staff. The nurse helps the CNA to understand this behavior by indicating that it most likely represents:
   1. a rejection of American culture by the client.
   2. a dislike of American school systems and the standard English language.
   3. a means of maintaining cultural identity.
   4. a permanent learning disability due to uncertain socioeconomic background.

33. Using knowledge of the family/social structure of the African-American culture, the nurse places highest priority on accommodating visits to Mrs. Haygood by which of the following individuals?
   1. Religious leader
   2. Local politician
   3. A new coworker
   4. A friend of a cousin

TEST YOURSELF

34. Which of the following is not a characteristic shared by people within an ethnic group?
   1. Religious faith or faiths
   2. External perception of distinctiveness
   3. Food preferences
   4. Loose or distant ties to others in the group

35. A culturally competent practitioner has which of the following attributes?
   1. Lack of awareness
   2. Sensitivity
   3. Lack of respect
   4. Ability to hold firm to one's viewpoint

Copyright © 2004, Elsevier Science (USA). All Rights Reserved.

36. A nurse who is speaking with a client from a different culture would find which of the following communication strategies to be least helpful?
    1. Asking the client about the meaning of health, illness, and planned care
    2. Finding out how the illness is likely to affect life, relationships, and self-concept
    3. Trying to anticipate the client's responses
    4. Asking the client how he or she prefers to manage the illness

37. A Mexican-American client tells the nurse about seeking the help of a *curandero* before coming to the health clinic. The nurse understands that, in the Mexican-American culture, this type of folk healer is a:
    1. holistic healer.
    2. healer who uses only herbs.
    3. male witch.
    4. female witch.

38. A hospitalized Chinese-American client states a preference for eating foods that have a yang quality. The nurse would offer the client which of the following food items?
    1. Cucumbers
    2. Oranges
    3. Watermelon
    4. Warm milk

Copyright © 2004, Elsevier Science (USA). All Rights Reserved.

The Health Care Delivery System

PURPOSE

As you begin your professional career in nursing, you will need to identify the components of the health care delivery system, identify the roles of members of the health care team, and understand the effects of social and political forces that will affect your practice. In this chapter you will be introduced to the providers, services, and financing methods that make up the health care delivery system in the United States. You will also explore some of the issues and opportunities facing health care delivery in the 21st century. You will want to further explore these issues as you learn more about health care delivery.

MATCHING

1. ____ access

2. ____ capitation payment system

3. ____ diagnosis-related group (DRG)

4. ____ exclusive provider organization (EPO)

5. ____ health maintenance organization (HMO)

6. ____ health promotion

7. ____ illness prevention

8. ____ managed care

9. ____ Medicaid

10. ____ Medicare

11. ____ preferred provider organization (PPO)

12. ____ prospective payment system

13. ____ rehabilitation

14. ____ retrospective payment system

   a. involves the use of immunizations and medications that avert disease or detect diseases in their earliest, most treatable stages

b. a complex construct representing the personal use of health care services and the structures or processes that facilitate or impede that use

c. a means to modify a client's knowledge, attitudes, and skills to adopt behaviors leading to a healthier lifestyle thus achieving a higher level of wellness from any point on a continuum from health to illness

d. a system of classification or grouping of patients according to medical diagnosis for purposes of paying hospitalization costs

e. a type of group health care practice in which enrollees are restricted to the list of preferred providers of health care, called "exclusive providers"

f. a type of group health care practice that provides basic and supplemental health maintenance and treatment services to voluntary enrollees who prepay a fixed periodic fee that is set without regard to the amount or kind of services received

g. payment for health care services is an arrangement between the purchaser of care and the provider in which the provider receives a flat fee to provide a defined level of care

h. has the goals of restoration of function, maintenance of the remaining levels of physical and mental function, and prevention of further deterioration

i. a system that combines the functions of health insurance and the actual delivery of care in a way that controls utilization and costs of services by limiting unnecessary treatment

j. a grant program providing partial health care services for indigent people; supported jointly by federal and state governments

k. a federally funded national health insurance program in the United States for people over 65 years of age and some chronically ill persons

Copyright © 2004, Elsevier Science (USA). All Rights Reserved.

l. an organization of physicians, hospitals, and pharmacists whose members discount their health care services to subscribers (clients); may be organized by a group of physicians, an outside entrepreneur, an insurance company, or a company with a self-insurance plan

m. a payment system in which what will be paid for, for a specific service, is predetermined

n. traditional method of reimbursement; insurance paid based on the services that are received

TRUE OR FALSE

15. ____ Nurses are the largest single group of health care professionals in the United States.

16. ____ Advanced nurse practitioners include nurse practitioners and physician assistants.

17. ____ Alternative practitioners are irrelevant to a discussion of health practices in the United States.

18. ____ Because of the strict regulation of hospitals, all Americans have equal access to high-quality hospital services.

19. ____ Long-term care (LTC) describes a range of health and housing services provided to people unable to care for themselves independently or in need of assistance to maintain their independence.

20. ____ Emergency medical technicians are trained to provide critical early treatment both on site and in transit, thus reducing the death rates from accidents and acute illness.

21. ____ Respite care is potentially cost effective because it helps those who need long-term care to stay at home.

22. ____ The U.S. government has only a limited role in the financing of health care.

23. ____ A health maintenance organization is a means of financing health care for its members but has no influence on the quality of care provided.

24. ____ Health care rationing is associated only with countries that have a national health care system.

25. ____ The fastest growing segment of the population is people over the age of 85.

26. ____ There will be a growing demand for health care providers who speak languages other than English and who understand the health needs of a multiethnic society.

27. ____ More than 13% of the U.S. gross national product is consumed by health care.

28. ____ As a nurse you will be primarily be concerned with quality of care rather than with cost of care.

FILL-IN-THE-BLANKS

29. Improvement in general health over the past few decades can be attributed to _____ and _____ .

30. _____ are the largest group of health care professionals in the United States.

31. _____ dispense medications and assist physicians in making appropriate drug choices.

32. The term _____ describes a client who receives care in the context of an overnight stay in a hospital or other health care facility.

33. An example of a first tier of the hospital system that offers more limited scope of services is a _____ .

34. _____ is a long-term-care service offered to clients who need restorative services or treatment to recover from an injury or illness.

35. _____ is a method of care that regards both the client and the family as the unit of care.

36. A _____ is the primary site for the delivery of physician services.

37. _____ is a daytime community-based program offered in an institutional setting that provides a wide range of health and recreational services to frail (usually elderly) adults who require supervision and care while members of the family are away at work.

38. The _____ spends more money per person on health care than any other country in the developed world.

39. A _____ may be organized by a group of physicians, an outside entrepreneur, an insurance company, or a company with a self-insurance plan.

40. Medicare finances health care for _____ , _____ , and _____ .

41. In _____ (country) the government finances health care, but private providers deliver health care services.

42. _____ percent of American households with children under the age of 18 include a married couple.

Copyright © 2004, Elsevier Science (USA). All Rights Reserved.

43. The _____ is a political action group that lobbies Congress with the hope of influencing legislation that affects older Americans.

EXERCISING YOUR CLINICAL JUDGMENT

You are working on a cardiac unit in a community hospital. Your client is a 58-year-old male who has had a minor heart attack. You are working with this person to plan for care after discharge. The following questions address the needs you and the client have identified.

44. The client has smoked a pack of cigarettes a day for 42 years. He knows he needs to quit but has been unsuccessful despite multiple attempts. He wants to join a support group. Which source is most likely to provide access (financial support) to a support group?
    1. A preferred provider organization
    2. A health maintenance organization
    3. Catastrophic health insurance
    4. Medicare

45. Your client would like to try the cholesterol-reducing medication that has recently been advertised on television. You would suggest that he ask his:
    1. pharmacist.
    2. physician.
    3. respiratory therapist.
    4. managed care organization.

46. You identify several misconceptions about the low-fat diet that has been prescribed by the physician. You know that the client's insurance will pay for any of the following, so you would make a referral to:
    1. an herbalist.
    2. a physical therapist.
    3. a dietitian.
    4. a physician assistant.

47. The physician has recommended a cardiac rehabilitation program for the next 6 months. You are reviewing a pamphlet about the program with the client. He asks, "What does rehabilitation mean? I thought that was for people who were paralyzed." Your best answer would be:
    1. "Rehabilitation is any long-term-care service for people who need additional therapy or treatment to recover from an illness or injury."
    2. "Using that term is a way to get your insurance to pay for the services."
    3. "Rehabilitation only refers to the exercise program that will be designed by a physical therapist."
    4. "Any service outside a hospital is rehabilitation."

TEST YOURSELF

48. Your client is being discharged after having a growth removed from her abdomen. The doctor has assured her that the tumor was benign and that no further treatment is indicated. She says, "My neighbor uses an Ayurveda practitioner. She had cancer 15 years ago and it has never returned. What do you think?" Your most appropriate response would be:
    1. "It sounds like a good idea to me. You never know what will work."
    2. "I don't think it's safe to use alternative medicine. None of it is proven."
    3. "You should learn more about it before trying it. Let me get you a pamphlet that gives some suggestions for evaluation of alternative practices."
    4. "Ayurveda therapy won't prevent the recurrence of cancer. You need to stick with your medical doctor."

49. Your client tells you that his insurance company will allow him to see any physician he chooses, but the fees are better if he chooses a physician from a list provided by the insurance company. He is most likely describing:
    1. a health maintenance organization.
    2. a managed care organization.
    3. Medicaid coverage.
    4. a preferred provider organization.

50. If you could make a change in the delivery of health care for the growing number of Hispanic-Americans, which would be most likely to result in integrating cost control and improved quality?
    1. Targeting genetically transmitted diseases that only affect Hispanics
    2. Increasing the number of Hispanic health providers
    3. Ensuring access to health care for Hispanic people
    4. Targeting the most common health problems for Hispanic people

51. A 95-year-old man is admitted to a nursing home after an episode of heart failure. Though the doctor has given him the option to have a heart valve replacement, the man has decided he prefers conservative treatment. The nursing home will monitor his medication and will help him achieve a balance of rest and activity, maintain a low-salt diet, and maintain his relationship with his family. This type of care is best labeled:
    1. illness prevention.
    2. acute care.
    3. rehabilitation.
    4. supportive care.

Copyright © 2004, Elsevier Science (USA). All Rights Reserved.

Caring and Clinical Judgment

5

PURPOSE

This chapter provides an understanding of the importance of nursing theory. It compares and contrasts the leading nursing theories, including the concepts of person, environment, health, and nursing are the most recognized organizing realities of nursing theory. Recently, nurse scientists have added caring to this group of concepts. It helps you learn to recognize the skills you use in thinking and when you are using different skills, and thus be able to improve the use of your thinking skills. It also introduces the nursing process, a patterned way of thinking used in making nursing judgments, decisions, and diagnoses. You will be able to identify how multiple thinking strategies apply to each phase of the nursing process.

MATCHING

1. ____ caring
2. ____ clinical judgment
3. ____ concept
4. ____ critical thinking
5. ____ decision making
6. ____ diagnostic reasoning
7. ____ empirical
8. ____ nursing process
9. ____ problem solving
10. ____ theory

   a. the process of clustering assessment data into meaningful sets and generating hypotheses about the client's human responses

   b. a critical thinking framework that includes decision making, diagnostic reasoning, problem solving, and clinical judgment; it is composed of five interrelated parts: assessment, diagnosis, planning, intervention, and evaluation

   c. defining a problem, selecting information pertinent to its conclusion (recognizing stated and unstated assumptions), formulating alternative solutions, drawing a conclusion, and judging the validity of the conclusion.

   d. purposeful self-regulatory judgment that gives reasoned and reflective consideration to evidence, contexts, conceptualizations, methods, and criteria

   e. choosing between two or more options as a means to achieve a desired result

   f. a conclusion or an opinion that a problem or situation requires nursing care

   g. a group of propositions used to describe, explain, or predict a phenomenon

   h. creative and rigorous structuring of ideas that project a tentative, purposeful, and systematic view of phenomena

   i. concepts that can be observed or experienced through the senses

   j. varies among cultures in its processes and patterns, is largely culturally derived, and is culturally expressed

TRUE OR FALSE

11. ____ Nursing theory can be of several different types.
12. ____ Theories are important to nurses because they interpret and explain the reality of nursing, thus guiding practice, education, and research activities for nursing as a profession.
13. ____ A nursing theory is unacceptable when the consensus of the nursing profession is that the theory provides an adequate description of reality.
14. ____ Roy believed that caring is the central theme in nursing knowledge and practice.
15. ____ The T.H.I.N.K. model is based on the idea that you use different elements of thinking in different situations.

Copyright © 2004, Elsevier Science (USA). All Rights Reserved.

16. ____ Inquiry includes the quality of being curious or wondering about the meaning of information.
17. ____ Routines in health care facilities are antithetical to critical thinking.
18. ____ Assessment means collecting answers to a predetermined list of questions.

FILL-IN-THE-BLANKS

19. The concepts of _____, environment, health, and _____ are the most recognized organizing realities of nursing theory.

20. It is helpful for you to know more than one nursing _____ because what you observe, document, choose as an intervention, and evaluate depends on your theoretical perspective guiding nursing practice.

21. Orem's theory focuses on the role of the _____ in helping clients meet their needs.

22. Obstacles to critical thinking include _____ _____ _____ _____ _____and _____.

23. In the planning phase you set _____ and plan _____ care.

24. Dependent interventions are those activities carried out under a _____ order.

25. NANDA stands for the _____ _____ _____ _____ _____.

TEST YOURSELF

26. Your client is Irish-American and has had abdominal surgery. You recognize the client's pain and her minimizing of the pain may be related to cultural ways. You stress to the client that if she has adequate pain relief she will be able to tend to all of her needs. You are applying which nursing theorist's theory?
    1. Hildegarde Peplau
    2. Faye Abdellah
    3. Dorothea Orem
    4. Madeleine Leininger

27. You are taking an admission history. You know the medical diagnosis but the client's report of symptoms does not exactly fit the pattern of expected symptoms. Which action would be the least consistent with critical thinking?
    1. Explore the symptoms further.
    2. Record the symptoms as described by the client.
    3. Record only the symptoms you believe are pertinent to the diagnosis.
    4. Ask the client about his perception of the symptoms.

28. You are starting a new job as a home health nurse. You must perform a procedure in the client's home. Although you have done the procedure many times in the hospital, you do not have the same resources in the home. Which mode of thinking will be the most useful to you?
    1. Total recall
    2. Habit
    3. Inquiry
    4. New ideas

29. A client complains of nausea. You know the physician has written an order for a medication to treat nausea if the client needs it. Using the nursing process to guide your thinking you would first:
    1. ask the client to further describe the nausea.
    2. give the antinausea medication.
    3. plan to cancel the client's lunch.
    4. notify the physician.

30. Nursing theories do which of the following?
    1. Differentiate the focus of nursing from other professions and are necessary for the continued growth and development of our profession
    2. Provide a conceptual diagram of the profession
    3. Are beliefs about phenomena
    4. Are relationship statements that are tested

31. Which nursing leader's theory is the primary basis for psychiatric nursing?
    1. Virginia Henderson
    2. Hildegarde Peplau
    3. Faye Abdellah
    4. Dorothea Orem

32. Which of the following nursing leaders emphasized that nursing is not something a person does, but a body of abstract knowledge and a learned profession that is both science and art?
    1. Virginia Henderson
    2. Hildegarde Peplau
    3. Faye Abdellah
    4. Martha Rogers

33. You assess your client and find sluggish skin turgor, sunken eyeballs, and a low urinary output. You know these are signs of dehydration and conclude that your client should drink more water. You have:
    1. made an interpretation of data.
    2. made an assumption.
    3. engaged in problem solving.
    4. recognized the purpose of thinking.

Copyright © 2004, Elsevier Science (USA). All Rights Reserved.

34. You are assigned to work with a staff nurse. The two of you enter a client's room and find the client slumped in bed. You assume the client is sleeping, but the staff nurse puts on the call light and picks up the phone to page for a resuscitation team. Which of Benner's stages apply to the staff nurse?
    1. Advanced beginner
    2. Competent
    3. Proficient
    4. Expert

35. You are assigned to a different nurse on the following day. A client tells you she does not need a laxative. The nurse tells you a laxative is always given after the procedure the client has had and you should insist the client take the laxative. This nurse is most likely in which stage?
    1. Novice
    2. Advanced beginner
    3. Competent
    4. Proficient

Copyright © 2004, Elsevier Science (USA). All Rights Reserved.

Client Assessment: Nursing History

PURPOSE

This chapter outlines the thinking skills associated with assessment and introduces a general pattern for taking a nursing history. You will learn additional information about nursing history with each clinical chapter you study.

MATCHING

1. ____ active listening
2. ____ active processing
3. ____ assessment
4. ____ biographical data
5. ____ cardinal signs and symptoms
6. ____ chief complaint
7. ____ closed question
8. ____ cue
9. ____ data
10. ____ database
11. ____ demographic data
12. ____ functional health patterns
13. ____ inference
14. ____ interview
15. ____ intuition
16. ____ leading question
17. ____ minimum data set
18. ____ nursing history
19. ____ objective data
20. ____ open-ended question
21. ____ orientation phase
22. ____ signs
23. ____ subjective data
24. ____ symptoms
25. ____ validation
26. ____ working phase

a. a phase of the interview process during which the client and nurse work together to review the client's health history and establish potential and actual problems that will be addressed as part of the care plan

b. subjective information that is indicative of disease as perceived by the client

c. substantiating or confirming the accuracy of the information against another source or by another method

d. information that is provided by the client and cannot be directly observed

e. the problem that caused the person to seek health services, to call the doctor, or to request a visit from the nurse; a description of what the person thinks is the problem

f. a planned series of questions designed to elicit information for a particular purpose

g. any directly observable information about the client

h. the positive and negative behaviors a person uses to interact with the environment and maintain health

i. a question designed to allow the client freedom in the manner of response

j. a process of reasoning from understanding the whole without having systematically examined the parts

Copyright © 2004, Elsevier Science (USA). All Rights Reserved.

k. a brief exchange to establish the purpose, the procedure, and the nurse's role as a phase of the interview process

l. objective data that are evidence of disease or dysfunction

m. a narrative of the client's past health and health practices that focuses on information needed to plan nursing care

n. the least information allowable to be collected on every client entering an institution or being admitted to a particular service within the institution

o. the process of attaching meaning to data or reaching a conclusion about data; based on a premise or proposition that supports or helps support a conclusion

p. question that suggests a possible appropriate response

q. information that identifies and describes the person, such as name, address, age, gender, religious affiliation, race, or occupation

r. question that calls for a specific response from the client

s. all of the information that has been collected about the client and recorded in the health record as a baseline for the initial plan of care

t. factual information that can be counted to describe populations of clients

u. the data of greatest significance in diagnosing a particular illness, disease, or health problem

v. a stimulus to the action of looking for related data

w. participation in a conversation with a client in which the nurse attends to what the client says and has a part in helping the client clarify, elaborate, and give additional pertinent information

x. the process of gathering data about the client's health status to identify the concerns and needs that can be treated or managed by nursing care

y. pieces of subjective or objective information about the client or the signs and symptoms of disease

z. a systematic series of mental actions to analyze and interpret information about the client

TRUE OR FALSE

27. ____ When prevention is the focus of care, client assessment includes risk and lifestyle factors.

28. ____ When, how often, and how to assess a client is a nursing judgment based on individual client needs.

29. ____ It is always appropriate to gather data from the client's family.

30. ____ Collecting data in a systematic way is a standard of nursing practice.

31. ____ Grouping data into meaningful patterns helps you translate the data into a meaningful statement.

32. ____ For any client, the purpose of an admission interview is always to collect a standard set of data.

33. ____ The termination phase of an interview is limited to the last few minutes of the interview.

34. ____ Biographical data are collected only to help you know the client as a person.

35. ____ The medical history is not part of the nursing history.

36. ____ Beliefs about health and about the ability to change health are a key element of the health perception–health management pattern.

37. ____ A functional health pattern includes both functional and dysfunctional patterns.

38. ____ The activity-exercise pattern includes only the musculoskeletal system.

39. ____ Only objective data are documented in the medical record.

40. ____ It is legally advisable to document the facts that lead to a conclusion or opinion rather than your own conclusion or opinion.

FILL-IN-THE-BLANKS

41. When the goal is _____, assessment focuses on the need for support of body functions and the detection and prevention of complications.

42. To decide how often to assess a client, you need to anticipate the _____, _____, and _____ of change.

43. The seven general factors used to assess a symptom are _____, _____, _____, _____, _____, _____ and _____, and _____.

44. _____implies a sense of understanding and trust between the nurse and client.

45. Questions describing the onset of symptoms, when symptoms occur, and the events surrounding symptoms are classified as _____.

46. A description of a client's dietary habits is included in the _____ - _____ pattern.

47. A description of a client's tolerance for activity is included in the _____ - _____ pattern.

Copyright © 2004, Elsevier Science (USA). All Rights Reserved.

48. A description of the client's perception of body image is included in the _____ - _____ / _____ - _____ pattern.

TEST YOURSELF

49. A female client who has four children, works full time, and volunteers in her church is admitted. She has peptic ulcer disease, an illness that is sometimes exacerbated by stress. In assessing the coping-stress tolerance pattern you would do which of the following?
    1. Assume the illness is exacerbated by stress.
    2. Plan to teach the client stress reduction techniques.
    3. Avoid discussion of the many stressors in the client's life.
    4. Validate the client's experience of stress by eliciting information about the client's perceptions.

50. You would assess the self-concept pattern on every client by doing which of the following activities?
    1. Asking a series of questions to elicit information about the self-concept
    2. Observing, listening, and being sensitive to covert messages
    3. Administering a standardized test for self-concept
    4. Asking the person to rate his or her self-concept on a scale of 1 to 10

51. A 55-year-old male is hospitalized for heart disease. His doctor has suggested he needs to retire. Which functional health pattern would you explore to help him through this experience?
    1. Sexuality-reproductive pattern
    2. Role-relationship pattern
    3. Coping-stress tolerance pattern
    4. Sleep-rest pattern

52. You are taking an admission history. The client tells you that he has pain in his leg. Which question is most pertinent to his safety in the hospital?
    1. "How long have you had the pain?"
    2. "Where is it located?"
    3. "Do you have any difficulty walking?"
    4. "What aggravates the pain?"

53. Your client has requested pain medication. If you could only ask one question for further assessment, which would you choose?
    1. "Did the last pain medication relieve the pain?"
    2. "How long have you had the pain?"
    3. "What brought on the pain?"
    4. "Is your pain less than yesterday's pain?"

54. Select the statement that is true of assessment.
    1. Assessment means collecting data.
    2. Assessment includes analyzing data to determine the need for nursing care.
    3. Assessment does not include physical examination.
    4. Assessment is a separate activity from planning and implementing care.

55. Which of the following items provides the best description of the term "focused assessment"?
    1. Paying close attention to the client's needs
    2. Concentrating on an identified need and getting more information
    3. Identifying the client's needs
    4. Using the acronym F.O.C.U.S.

56. Which of the following items provides the best description of objective data?
    1. It is pertinent to an objective or goal.
    2. It can be gathered through the use of one of the five senses.
    3. It is elicited from the client in an objective manner.
    4. It relates to the objects in the client's room.

57. You are sharing information with the client's physician that the wife of your client has given you. The physician asks you if the wife is a reliable source. Which of the following data is the most useful to you in deciding that the wife is a reliable source?
    1. The couple has been arguing about the nature of his symptoms.
    2. The husband has told you to talk to his wife about his symptoms.
    3. The wife presents information factually and has kept a diary of the symptoms.
    4. The husband shows evidence of minor memory impairment.

58. *Fact:* Your client's antihypertensive medication prescription was filled 15 days ago with 60 tablets. He is supposed to take 2 tablets a day. He has 40 tablets left. *Premise:* There is a high incidence of failure to take blood pressure medications correctly among people with hypertension because of side effects. Select the most accurate conclusion.
    1. The client does not understand how to take the medication.
    2. The client does not want to take the medication.
    3. The client has taken the medication incorrectly.
    4. The side effects have been intolerable for the client.

Copyright © 2004, Elsevier Science (USA). All Rights Reserved.

Assessing Vital Signs

PURPOSE

The purpose of this chapter is to help you learn accurate techniques for measuring vital signs and to understand the physiological changes that affect vital signs. You will also begin the process of interpreting or attaching meaning to your findings.

MATCHING

1. ____ apical pulse
2. ____ auscultatory gap
3. ____ basal metabolic rate
4. ____ bradycardia
5. ____ bradypnea
6. ____ diastolic blood pressure
7. ____ eupnea
8. ____ hypertension
9. ____ hypotension
10. ____ Korotkoff's sounds
11. ____ pulse deficit
12. ____ pulse pressure
13. ____ systolic blood pressure
14. ____ tachypnea
15. ____ thermogenesis
16. ____ thermolysis

a. the condition of the apical pulse rate exceeding the radial pulse rate

b. the processes through which heat is dispersed from the body through radiation, conduction, convection, and evaporation expressed as calories per hour per square meter of body surface

c. the generation of heat from the chemical reactions that take place in cellular activity

d. the heart rate counted at the apex of the heart on the anterior chest

e. the amount of energy needed to maintain essential basic body functions expressed as calories per hour per square meter of body surface

f. the difference between the systolic and diastolic pressure

g. normal quiet respiration

h. the absence of Korotkoff II sounds; sometimes present in hypertension

i. a heart rate insufficient to produce adequate tissue perfusion (when it continues over a long time), usually less than 60

j. a respiratory rate insufficient to take in enough oxygen (when it continues over a long time), usually below 10

k. the pressure in the blood vessels that remains during relaxation of the ventricles

l. generally defined as a blood pressure greater than 140/90

m. generally defined as a blood pressure below 100/60

n. five distinct sounds heard as a blood pressure cuff is deflated from total occlusion of the artery to complete free flow of blood

o. the pressure in the arteries produced by the cardiac output during contraction of the ventricle

p. rapid respiration

TRUE OR FALSE

17. ____ The absolute value of vital signs is the basis for inferences about vital signs.

18. ____ How often you take vital signs is a nursing judgment.

Copyright © 2004, Elsevier Science (USA). All Rights Reserved.

19. ____ The body's cells work within a narrow range of normal temperature but can tolerate some changes for a brief period.

20. ____ High temperatures damage cells by inactivating proteins and enzymes.

21. ____ An oral temperature can be accurately measured by placing the thermometer anywhere in the mouth.

22. ____ Clean a glass thermometer by wiping from the bulb toward the end.

23. ____ A heart rate of 100 is always a cause for concern.

24. ____ Vomiting can cause bradycardia.

25. ____ Adrenalin increases the heart rate.

26. ____ Head injuries always cause the heart rate to increase.

27. ____ The strength of the pulse wave is only a function of the strength of myocardial contraction.

28. ____ The carotid artery is the most common site for counting the pulse.

29. ____ The most accurate pulse count is obtained at the apex of the heart.

30. ____ The medullary control center for respiration responds to high levels of carbon dioxide.

31. ____ Sighing is a protective mechanism that periodically expands unused alveoli.

FILL-IN-THE-BLANKS

32. _____ _____ are the signs of life.

33. The processes through which the body balances heat production and heat loss to maintain a temperature between 96.8° F and 99.4° F is called _____.

34. The _____ thermometer is inexpensive, accurate, and easily disinfected; however, it may be difficult to read for some clients in their homes.

35. The _____ thermometer is accurate if the probe is directed on the eardrum.

36. Children have a slightly higher heart rate than adults do because they have a higher _____ _____.

37. Adrenergic drugs (acting like adrenaline) will cause the heart rate to _____ (increase, decrease).

38. When the pulse wave increases during inhalation and decreases back to normal during exhalation, the phenomenon is called _____ _____.

39. When blood vessels constrict, blood flow is impeded because the lumen of the vessels is smaller. The smaller diameter creates peripheral vascular _____.

40. The systolic blood pressure is created by the _____ (contraction, relaxation) of the ventricles.

41. The diastolic blood pressure is the pressure that remains during _____ (contraction, relaxation) of the ventricles.

42. The width of the blood pressure cuff should be about _____ _____ the length of the upper arm.

TEST YOURSELF

43. Your client has a temperature of 103° F, respirations of 30, pulse of 50. She is cold and clammy and her blood pressure is 100/60. Which conclusion is most consistent with these findings?
    1. The temperature has caused a decrease in her pulse rate. Correcting the temperature will fix the problem.
    2. The low pulse is causing a decrease in cardiac output, thus reducing the blood pressure. It may or may not be related to the temperature.
    3. The low pulse and blood pressure is a compensatory response to decrease the metabolic rate.
    4. The high temperature is consistent with the low pulse and blood pressure.

44. The physician tells you that the client has atherosclerotic vascular disease that is increasing peripheral vascular resistance. Which vital signs would be consistent with this information?
    1. Blood pressure 140/100, pulse 90, respiration 18
    2. Blood pressure 110/60, pulse 60, respiration 18
    3. Blood pressure 160/80, pulse 56, respiration 16
    4. Blood pressure 140/84, pulse 80, respiration 20

45. Your client's blood pressure (BP) is 180/106. You administer an antihypertensive drug and come to the room to recheck the BP in 1 hour. You find the client in the bathroom and she is pale, sweating, and feels faint. You get her back to bed and take her vital signs. Which would you expect?
    1. BP 180/106; the medication did not work.
    2. BP 120/80; the sudden drop caused the symptoms.
    3. BP 160/96; the medication is taking effect, but has made her sick.
    4. BP 120/80; the medication has been effective, and the symptoms have another cause.

Copyright © 2004, Elsevier Science (USA). All Rights Reserved.

46. Digitalis is a medication that slows the heart rate and strengthens the contraction. Before giving digitalis it is a common practice to check the pulse. If the client's pulse has been averaging 80 for the last 3 days, which pulse rate would suggest that the expected result has become a toxic effect?
    1. Pulse 56
    2. Pulse 66
    3. Pulse 76
    4. Pulse 96

47. Your client was burned on the right arm while lighting a charcoal fire. He has an intravenous line in the left arm that was inserted with difficulty. Which action would you take related to vital signs?
    1. Because he is awake and alert, omit taking a blood pressure.
    2. Use a smaller size cuff for the blood pressure.
    3. Take the blood pressure in the thigh.
    4. Assess the systolic pressure only by palpating the radial artery.

48. You have admitted a 16-month-old with fever of unknown origin. The child's cheeks are red and the skin feels warm to the touch. The tympanic thermometer reads 98.6° F. Which of the following would be the best action?
    1. Check the temperature in the room and lower the thermostat for comfort.
    2. Ask the mother about the technique she used to take the temperature to determine if the reported fever was accurate.
    3. Straighten the ear canal and recheck the temperature. Use another method if necessary to accurately measure the temperature.
    4. Recalibrate the thermometer and check the temperature.

49. You take a client's temperature at 6 am. It is 96.8° F. What is the most probable cause?
    1. A cold room
    2. Drinking ice water
    3. Circadian rhythms
    4. A faulty thermometer

50. Which of the following activities is appropriate when preparing to take an axillary temperature?
    1. Dry the axilla before inserting the thermometer.
    2. Lubricate the thermometer before insertion.
    3. Position patient in the side-lying position.
    4. Shave the axilla.

51. The client's rectal temperature is 100° F. After conversion, which of the following would be the comparable axillary temperature?
    1. 97° F
    2. 98° F
    3. 99° F
    4. 101° F

52. Which of the following is the primary reason you should avoid taking a blood pressure on the same arm with an intravenous infusion?
    1. The blood pressure will be inaccurate.
    2. Blood from the IV line will contaminate the blood pressure cuff.
    3. The increased venous pressure will cause blood to back up in the IV tubing.
    4. The blood pressure reading will be higher.

53. Nurses have some discretion in selecting the route to take a temperature. Which of the following represents the best judgment?
    1. Taking an oral temperature in a 12-month-old child
    2. Taking a rectal temperature in a confused 85-year-old man
    3. Taking an axillary temperature in a newborn
    4. Taking an oral temperature on a client who had oral surgery

54. Select the situation that may result in an inaccurate measurement of blood pressure.
    1. The width of cuff is 20% greater than the diameter of arm.
    2. The aneroid sphygmomanometer is viewed from the side.
    3. The meniscus of the mercury manometer is at eye level.
    4. The cuff is placed 1 inch above the fold of the elbow.

55. Which of the following should be recorded as the diastolic pressure in an adult?
    1. The first distinct beat that is heard
    2. The change in sound from a clear distinct tapping to a soft muffled sound
    3. The middle sound between the first and last beat heard
    4. The last sound that is heard

56. To obtain the most accurate blood pressure reading the cuff should be inflated to:
    1. 20 to 30 mm Hg above the palpated systolic pressure.
    2. the systolic reading last recorded on the client's chart.
    3. 50 mm Hg above the last diastolic reading.
    4. 200 mm Hg in an adult client,

57. Which action might result in a falsely low systolic blood pressure reading?
    1. Allowing the client to cross the legs while BP is being taken
    2. Deflating the cuff too rapidly while BP is being auscultated.
    3. Requiring the client to support the arm isometrically while BP is being taken
    4. Having the client think relaxing thoughts

Copyright © 2004, Elsevier Science (USA). All Rights Reserved.

58. Select the inference that is most accurate without further assessment.
    1. A right radial pulse of 88 beats/minute indicates that the person has adequate oxygenation to the right hand.
    2. Respirations of 18 per minute indicate that the person is taking in sufficient amounts of oxygen.
    3. The auscultated blood pressure of 130/88 is a normal blood pressure for this particular person.
    4. When the apical pulse is 80 and the radial pulse is 60, the client has a pulse deficit.

59. A client is admitted to the hospital with an irregular pulse of 110. Which of the following would be the best method to use to further evaluate the pulse?
    1. Take an apical-radial pulse and subtract the difference.
    2. Subtract the difference between the right and left radial pulses.
    3. Count the time it takes for an apical beat to reach the radial pulses.
    4. Count the number of irregular beats to determine a pulse deficit.

60. A client has just been admitted with a lung infection. His vital signs indicate hypotension, tachycardia, and tachypnea. This information would be supported by which set of data?
    1. BP 150/105, pulse 123, respirations 12
    2. BP 90/40, pulse 110, respirations 28
    3. BP 120/80, pulse 50, respirations 40
    4. BP 115/80, pulse 100, respirations 30

61. A client had a temperature of 104° F at 10 am. At 1 pm the skin is warm and wet with perspiration. The nurse retakes the temperature. Select the finding that would be expected.
    1. A normal or near-normal temperature is found.
    2. The fever has not abated.
    3. The temperature has increased.
    4. The client is anxious.

62. For which of the following clients would you take a rectal rather than an oral temperature?
    1. A 10-year-old girl admitted with a urinary tract infection
    2. A 79-year-old man with dentures who is NPO for surgery
    3. A 40-year-old male admitted for new onset confusion
    4. An 80-year-old female admitted for a total hip replacement

63. A 45-year-old client has been in a motor vehicle accident (MVA). He was examined in the emergency room and transferred to your unit for observation. Vital signs are BP 100/60, P 94, R 22, and T 98.6° F. Select the best conclusion concerning these findings.
    1. The vital signs may indicate impending shock; notify the physician.
    2. These are normal findings for this age; continue routine monitoring.
    3. These may be normal findings, but there is concern about the BP; continue monitoring.
    4. He probably received pain medication in the emergency room.

Copyright © 2004, Elsevier Science (USA). All Rights Reserved.

Physical Assessment

PURPOSE

This chapter provides information about the basic techniques of physical examination and provides the basis to assist you in being able to identify normal findings. You will also be introduced to some abnormal findings as a way to help you begin to compare normal and abnormal findings.

MATCHING

1. ____ auscultation

2. ____ bronchial

3. ____ bronchovesicular

4. ____ ecchymosis

5. ____ inspection

6. ____ lesion

7. ____ ophthalmoscope

8. ____ otoscope

9. ____ palpation

10. ____ percussion

11. ____ precordium

12. ____ point of maximum impulse

13. ____ turgor

14. ____ vesicular

   a. the area on the anterior chest overlying the heart and great vessels

   b. the use of short, sharp strikes to the body surface to produce palpable vibrations and characteristic sounds

   c. a form of touch or feeling with the hand; it is used to obtain information regarding temperature, moisture, texture, consistency, size, shape, position, and movement

   d. normal breath sounds that occur between sounds of the bronchial tubes and those of the alveoli, or a combination of the two sounds

   e. the process of listening to sounds generated within the body

   f. a normal sound heard with a stethoscope over the main airways, including trachea and sternum

   g. the systematic visual examination of the client

   h. a wound, injury, or pathological change in the body

   i. an instrument used to visualize the retina, including the optic disk, macula, and retinal blood vessels through the pupil

   j. an instrument used to examine the external ear, the eardrum, and, through the eardrum, the ossicles of the middle ear; consists of a light, a magnifying lens, a speculum, and sometimes a device for insufflation

   k. the point where the heart comes the closest to the chest wall at the apex of the heart

   l. a reflection of the skin's elasticity measured as the time it takes for the skin to return to normal after being pinched lightly between the thumb and forefinger

   m. a normal sound of rustling or swishing heard with a stethoscope over the lung periphery, characteristically higher pitched during inspiration and falling rapidly during expiration

   n. a blue-black skin discoloration characterized by large irregularly formed hemorrhagic areas that changes to greenish brown or yellow during healing

TRUE OR FALSE

15. ____ A good quality stethoscope has a thin wall.

16. ____ A stethoscope amplifies sounds to enable you to hear.

Copyright © 2004, Elsevier Science (USA). All Rights Reserved.

17. ____ You should always begin the physical examination with the client in the sitting position.

18. ____ The sagittal plane divides the body into right and left halves.

19. ____ The heart is located lateral to the midline on the right side.

20. ____ The advantage of balanced scale is accuracy because the scale can be balanced at zero with each use.

21. ____ If the client can tell you that the current time of day is after lunchtime, you may assume orientation to time.

22. ____ Damage to the facial nerve (cranial nerve VII) results in lack of control of the muscles needed to close the eye.

23. ____ Yearly eye exams are indicated for people with bleeding disorders or those on anticoagulant therapy.

24. ____ PERRLA is checked on the unconscious client to determine visual acuity.

25. ____ Arteries are distinguishable as brighter than veins when checking the ocular fundus.

26. ____ You should angle the otoscope at a 90-degree angle to the ear to visualize the eardrum.

27. ____ The thyroid gland should feel smooth and hard.

28. ____ A cervical lymph node that is less than 1 cm with definite margins, and is mobile and nontender, is a normal finding.

29. ____ Assessing the breast for lumps includes assessing the axilla.

30. ____ The upper lobe of the right lung is assessed above an imaginary line from the posterior fold of the axilla to the midaxillary line at the sixth rib.

31. ____ Decreased respiratory excursion occurs with any condition that limits the expansion of the lungs.

32. ____ S_2 is associated with the closure of the pulmonic and aortic valves.

33. ____ An apical/radial pulse should be checked on every client with heart disease.

34. ____ A rapid rhythm with an S_3 sound is described as a ventricular gallop.

35. ____ A grade 6 murmur is barely audible.

36. ____ A bruit is normally heard at the carotid artery because of the vessel's large size.

37. ____ If you cannot feel a popliteal pulse you should confirm its absence with a Doppler.

38. ____ Identifying hypoactive bowel sounds is a precise measurement of the volume and frequency of the sounds.

39. ____ A gastric bubble causes a tympanic sound with percussion over the right upper quadrant.

40. ____ The Babinski reflex should be absent in an adult.

FILL-IN-THE-BLANKS

41. Use the technique of _____ _____ to identify and examine lesions or masses on the surface of the skin or immediately under the skin.

42. Use the physical assessment skill of _____ to tap on the abdomen to detect the presence of "gas" or flatus.

43. Using the technique of listening to the abdomen is called _____.

44. _____ _____ refers to patterns of thinking such as logic, relevance, organization, and coherence of thought.

45. Skin is best assessed in _____ light.

46. _____ is a crackling or rubbing sound heard during movement of joints, such as the temporomandibular joint.

47. A reported result of 30/60–2 on a visual acuity test means the person is able to read with _____ errors at a distance of _____ feet, a line of print that a person with normal vision could read at _____ feet.

48. The _____ test is a hearing test that compares air and bone conduction using a tuning fork.

49. In periodontal disease the client often has red, swollen gums indicating _____.

50. _____ respiration is the deep rapid breathing seen in diabetic ketoacidosis.

51. If you hear an abnormal breath sound in part of the cycle of respiration (such as with inspiration and not expiration) you would describe the sound as _____ (continuous, discontinuous).

52. _____ _____ reflexes are elicited by stretching a tendon by tapping with a reflex hammer.

53. The _____ _____ is a cytology test to screen for cervical cancer.

Copyright © 2004, Elsevier Science (USA). All Rights Reserved.

54. The _____ gland encircles the male urethra.

55. A _____ can be felt as a string of beadlike nodules or "bag of worms" in the scrotum.

TEST YOURSELF

56. Your client is a 90-year-old who is admitted to the hospital with a respiratory problem. She seems clean, well groomed, and well nourished but is unsteady when walking, seems a little confused, and has pain in her chest. Circle all of the elements of the physical exam that you would consider essential.
    1. Assess for adventitious sounds
    2. Formal mental status exam
    3. Assess all pulses
    4. Complete abdominal assessment
    5. Rectal examination
    6. Skin assessment
    7. Complete musculoskeletal assessment
    8. Inspection of the toenails
    9. Hearing and vision screening
    10. Assess the rate and rhythm of the heart
    11. Listen for murmurs

57. Your client has returned from a cardiac catheterization. The catheter was threaded through the right femoral artery. You are checking for blood clots traveling from the artery to the lower leg. The dorsalis pedis pulse is strong. What would you do next?
    1. Check the popliteal pulse.
    2. Check the femoral pulse.
    3. Check the color and warmth of the toes.
    4. Conclude that the circulation is good.

58. Your client has an irregular heartbeat and the apical/radial pulse is 80/60. Which of the following additional findings you would expect?
    1. Talkative, color pink, looking forward to visitors
    2. Blood pressure low, skin pale, feels weak
    3. Skin hot, face flushed, feels anxious
    4. Mentally alert, BP 140/90, respiration 16

59. Which assessment data provide the nurse with the best information regarding the client's ability to perfuse distal tissues?
    1. Blood pressure, Homans' sign, and breath sounds
    2. Respirations, peripheral pulses, and skin turgor
    3. Capillary refill, peripheral pulses, and skin color
    4. Skin turgor, skin color, and quality of pulse

60. During lung auscultation, the nurse would ask the client to do which of the following?
    1. Breathe deeply with mouth open
    2. Cough with each inhalation
    3. Hold the breath
    4. Breathe quietly and normally

61. During assessment you cannot palpate the pedal pulses bilaterally. Which of the following would be the best nursing action to take next?
    1. Palpate the femoral arteries.
    2. Immediately call the doctor.
    3. Assess color and temperature of the client's feet.
    4. Ask the client to wiggle the toes.

62. A client's left radial pulse is assessed as irregular. Which of the following would be the best nursing action?
    1. Take an apical pulse for 1 full minute.
    2. Recount the radial pulse for 2 minutes to assess for regularity.
    3. Have another nurse check the right radial pulse while the first nurse recounts the left pulse.
    4. Record the finding without further assessment.

63. After auscultating a client's abdomen for 30 seconds, the nurse hears hypoactive bowel sounds in the RUQ and LUQ, and hears no bowel sounds in the RLQ and LLQ. Which of the following would be the best nursing action?
    1. Immediately report this information to the physician.
    2. Listen 1 to 3 minutes in each of the lower quadrants.
    3. Chart this information and reassess in 8 hours.
    4. Assess for abdominal distention.

64. When the nurse elicits calf pain on dorsiflexion of the client's right foot, which of the following represents the best documentation?
    1. Complains of cramping pain in right calf
    2. Positive Homans' sign right leg
    3. Painful right leg bruit
    4. Deep vein thrombosis

65. Your client is telling you about the difficult times he has had since the death of his wife. He is smiling and periodically interrupts his story with a giggle. You most likely use which of the following terms to describe his affect?
    1. Flat
    2. Inappropriate
    3. Nonplus
    4. Timorous

Copyright © 2004, Elsevier Science (USA). All Rights Reserved.

66. Your client's skin has a yellow cast and you observe yellow color of the conjunctiva. Which of the following terms would you use to document this finding?
    1. Cyanosis
    2. Flushing
    3. Normal
    4. Jaundice

67. You ask the client to smile, frown, raise the eyebrows, or tightly close the eyes. Which cranial nerve are you testing?
    1. I
    2. III
    3. V
    4. VII

68. When you ask a client to read a newspaper or pamphlet, you are testing which of the following?
    1. Distance vision
    2. Near vision
    3. Discrimination
    4. Accommodation

69. To check the ocular fundus, begin with the ophthalmoscope approximately how many inches from the eye?
    1. 5
    2. 10
    3. 15
    4. 20

70. When you palpate the sinuses you are primarily looking for which of the following?
    1. Changes in temperature
    2. Changes in color
    3. Tenderness
    4. Nodules

71. When examining the tonsils as part of an oropharyngeal assessment, you would expect to see which of the following?
    1. Tonsils somewhat darker than the rest of the oropharynx
    2. An irregular tonsillar surface
    3. Tonsils that do not protrude beyond the tonsillar pillar
    4. Tonsils that protrude between the pillars and the uvula

72. To palpate cervical lymph nodes, you feel on both sides of the neck at the same time. Which of the following represents the reason for this technique?
    1. To save time
    2. For bilateral comparison
    3. To prevent distortion
    4. To compress the neck

73. When you are assessing for breast symmetry you would expect to find which of the following?
    1. Both breasts have perfectly equal symmetry.
    2. The right breast is larger in right-handed people.
    3. The breasts have the same general shape, with some minor variation.
    4. The breasts are of equal size.

74. To detect excess mucus in the bifurcation of the bronchi you would listen in which of the following areas?
    1. At the third intercostal space on the right
    2. Over the sternum at the angle of Louis
    3. Over the sternum at the level of the fourth rib
    4. At the sternal angle

75. To assess the bases of the lungs you would listen posteriorly over which of the following areas?
    1. 12th intercostal space
    2. 10th intercostal space
    3. 8th intercostal space
    4. 6th intercostal space

76. The physician's physical examination report identifies a grade 3 holosystolic murmur. Which of the following would you expect to hear?
    1. A moderately loud muffled or nondistinct sound throughout S_1
    2. A moderately loud muffled or nondistinct sound throughout S_2
    3. A barely audible S_1 and S_2
    4. A barely audible muffled or nondistinct sound throughout S_2

77. Even if the client has liver disease, the liver is not assessed every shift or even daily. The rationale for this action is that:
    1. nurses can't legally perform liver assessment.
    2. it involves deep palpation, causing unnecessary discomfort.
    3. there are other better signs of liver enlargement.
    4. liver enlargement is a normal finding in many people.

78. Observing your client from the posterior, you notice an S-shaped curve to the spine. You would describe this finding as which of the following?
    1. Ankylosing spondylitis
    2. Lordosis
    3. Scoliosis
    4. Kyphosis

Copyright © 2004, Elsevier Science (USA). All Rights Reserved.

79. Screening for sexual abuse includes external inspection of the genitalia. In a 3-year-old female, you would be less suspicious of sexual abuse if you made which of the following observations about the hymen?
    1. It is edematous.
    2. It is intact.
    3. It is absent.
    4. It is torn.

80. Which of the following findings is associated with scrotal edema?
    1. Slightly darker pigmentation than the rest of the body
    2. Absence of rugae
    3. The left testicle is lower than the right
    4. Presence of a varicocele

Copyright © 2004, Elsevier Science (USA). All Rights Reserved.

Nursing Diagnosis

PURPOSE

This chapter provides information about the process of making a nursing diagnosis. It also provides an overview of nursing diagnosis classification systems, diagnostic reasoning, and preventing nursing diagnostic errors.

MATCHING

1. ____ clinical judgment

2. ____ collaborative problem

3. ____ cue

4. ____ defining characteristics

5. ____ descriptor

6. ____ diagnostic label

7. ____ diagnostic reasoning

8. ____ differential diagnosis

9. ____ nursing diagnosis

10. ____ related factors

11. ____ risk factors

12. ____ "risk for" nursing diagnosis

13. ____ taxonomy

14. ____ wellness nursing diagnosis

   a. a system of identification, naming, and classification of phenomena

   b. the name of the nursing diagnosis

   c. internal or external environmental factors that increase the vulnerability of a person, family, or community to an unhealthful event

   d. a process of logical, flexible thinking to solve problems and plan nursing care that accounts for individual client needs and uses the individual strengths of the client and nurse to the fullest

   e. those factors that appear to show some type of patterned relationship with the nursing diagnosis

   f. describes human responses that may develop in a vulnerable person, family, or community

   g. a conclusion or an opinion that a problem or situation requires nursing care and that determines the cause of the problem, distinguishes between similar problems, or discriminates among two or more courses of action

   h. an indicator of the presence or existence of a problem or condition that represents a client's underlying health status

   i. descriptors of a client's behavior that determine whether a nursing diagnosis is present and whether a particular diagnosis is appropriate or accurate

   j. a clinical problem that cannot be solved by the nursing staff alone, but requires medications or treatments that nurses are not licensed to order

   k. describes human responses to levels of wellness in an individual, family, or community with a potential for growth and/or enhancement to a higher state

   l. a clinical judgment about individual, family, or community responses to actual or potential health problems or life processes

   m. the process of deciding among several possible diagnoses to most accurately describe the client's problem

   n. a word, such as *impaired, decreased, ineffective, acute*, or *chronic*, that modifies or limits a nursing diagnosis, or gives it greater specificity

TRUE OR FALSE

15. ____ Nursing diagnosis is a problem for which nurses are accountable and can diagnose and treat independently.

Copyright © 2004, Elsevier Science (USA). All Rights Reserved.

16. ____ Nursing diagnosis is part of the nursing process.

17. ____ The American Nurses Association is the group that develops, refines, and promotes a taxonomy of nursing diagnoses.

18. ____ A benefit of nursing diagnosis is that it contributes to the autonomy and self-regulatory capacity of nursing.

19. ____ "Experiencing" is one of the nine NANDA patterns of response.

20. ____ A nursing diagnosis staged as Level 1 incorporates a diagnosis from the time it is recommended with a label until it is placed on the taxonomy list for study.

21. ____ A limitation of the current NANDA diagnosis group is that it does not adequately include wellness diagnoses, community health nursing diagnoses, or psychiatric diagnoses.

22. ____ A diagnostic label gives a nursing diagnosis greater specificity.

23. ____ The process of making a nursing diagnosis involves several interrelated steps.

24. ____ Nursing diagnoses should seldom, if ever, be discussed with the client.

FILL-IN-THE-BLANKS

25. Nursing diagnosis is the _____ phase of the nursing process.

26. The _____ System has developed from 15 years of research and includes nursing diagnoses that reflect the home and community health setting.

27. The first part of a nursing diagnostic statement is the _____ _____.

28. *Family coping: potential for growth* is an example of a _____ nursing diagnosis.

29. After gathering nursing assessment data, the nurse _____ it to gain insight into the client's condition.

30. The nurse who is engaged in the nursing diagnosis step of _____ among possible diagnoses is narrowing the number of possible nursing diagnoses to identify the most appropriate one.

31. A _____ _____ is a descriptor of a client's behavior that determines whether a nursing diagnosis is present and appropriate or accurate.

32. The nursing diagnosis *Ineffective infant feeding pattern related to negligent mothering and maternal selfishness* written in a client's chart could be viewed as _____ in a court of law.

33. Trying to include every possible nursing diagnosis that could ever apply to a client would be considered to be the nursing diagnosis error of _____.

EXERCISING YOUR CLINICAL JUDGMENT

Mrs. Marcus had her gallbladder removed in surgery earlier in the day, and has an incision in the right upper abdomen near the diaphragm. Her temperature is 98.8°F, pulse is 92, respirations 22/minute and shallow. Blood pressure is stable at 128/78 mm Hg. Mrs. Marcus has an intravenous line for fluid replacement and has an indwelling Foley catheter to drain urine from the bladder. She complains that it hurts to take a deep breath and exhibits guarding of the incision area. She says she feels "achy" from being immobilized on the operating room table. The last dose of a prn narcotic analgesic was given 3 hours ago and is now due. The nurse who admitted Mrs. Marcus from the postanesthesia care unit must formulate a list of nursing diagnoses and develop a plan of care.

34. Which of the following nursing diagnoses represents the most well-constructed nursing diagnostic statement about this client's pain?
   1. *Pain related to right upper abdominal incision and operative positioning*
   2. *Risk for pain related to frequency of ordered narcotic analgesic*
   3. *Pain related to insufficient pain medication frequency*
   4. *Risk for pain related to overall surgical experience*

35. If the nurse is considering the nursing diagnosis *Risk for urinary retention*, when should it be instituted?
   1. When the nurse writes the initial care plan
   2. When the Foley catheter is discontinued
   3. When the client's urine output falls below 30 mL/hour with the catheter in place
   4. When the client is ready for discharge to home

36. Which of the following would be the most appropriate nursing diagnosis for the client's respiratory status?
   1. *Risk for impaired gas exchange due to increased secretions*
   2. *Risk for ineffective breathing pattern related to subdiaphragmatic incision and guarding*
   3. *Ineffective airway clearance related to weak cough and shallow respirations*
   4. *Impaired gas exchange due to anesthesia and abnormal respiratory rate*

Copyright © 2004, Elsevier Science (USA). All Rights Reserved.

37. If the nurse considers the possibility that the client could develop an infection in the wound or because of invasive lines, the nursing diagnosis would be written as which of the following?
    1. An actual diagnosis
    2. A wellness diagnosis
    3. A medical diagnosis
    4. A "risk for" diagnosis

TEST YOURSELF

38. Which of the following is one of the limitations of the current NANDA system for classifying nursing diagnoses?
    1. It is specific to only a few nursing specialties.
    2. It is not well accepted in nursing education.
    3. It is endorsed by the American Nurses' Association.
    4. It contains diagnoses at different levels of abstraction.

39. The part of the nursing diagnostic statement that contains a descriptor is called:
    1. a diagnostic label.
    2. a definition.
    3. the defining characteristics.
    4. the etiologic factors.

40. Which of the following is the broadest and highest level type of thinking that may be required for clinical nursing practice?
    1. Ordinary, logical thinking
    2. Clinical judgment
    3. Critical thinking
    4. Diagnostic reasoning

41. A nurse working in a community health setting would choose which of the following nursing diagnoses as the most realistic after taking into consideration the care setting?
    1. Impaired home maintenance management
    2. Decreased cardiac output
    3. Ineffective thermoregulation
    4. Decreased adaptive capacity: intracranial

42. For which of the following reasons is the nursing diagnosis *Ineffective airway clearance related to infrequent suctioning* most inappropriate?
    1. It is judgmental.
    2. It is derogatory.
    3. It suggests negligence.
    4. It suggests poor opinion of colleagues.

Copyright © 2004, Elsevier Science (USA). All Rights Reserved.

Planning, Intervening, and Evaluating

PURPOSE

The purpose of this chapter is to introduce you to planning, intervention, and evaluation as phases of the nursing process. Although the chapter focuses on the individual, you will also consider planning, intervention, and evaluation for groups of clients who have a common set of needs. Planning and intervention are inherent parts of designing and delivering services to meet the needs of a client population. During evaluation you will measure expected client outcomes and determine the degree to which an institution's external and internal standards are met.

MATCHING

1. ____ case management
2. ____ clinical pathway
3. ____ discharge planning
4. ____ evaluation
5. ____ expected outcomes
6. ____ goal
7. ____ individualized care plan
8. ____ long-term goal
9. ____ nursing care plan
10. ____ nurse-initiated intervention
11. ____ nursing intervention
12. ____ Nursing Intervention Classification (NIC)
13. ____ Nursing Outcome Classification (NOC)
14. ____ nursing-sensitive client outcome
15. ____ physician-initiated intervention
16. ____ short-term goal

a. broad, general statements about the desired results of nursing care

b. a care delivery system that focuses on the management of client care across an episode of illness

c. a standardized language appropriate for computerized client information systems to describe the component of client care that is nursing practice

d. a measurable client or family caregiver state, behavior, or perception that is conceptualized as a variable and is largely influenced by nursing interventions

e. a systematic and ongoing process of examining whether expected outcomes have been achieved and whether nursing care has been effective

f. written separately for each client who enters a health care facility; allows for the nurse to identify the unique problems of each client to decide on the outcomes to be achieved and to identify which nursing interventions will be appropriate to achieve those outcomes

g. suggests that the resolution of the nursing diagnosis can be accomplished in a hour, day, or week

h. within the independent scope of nursing practice and prescribed by the nurse independent of the physician

i. within the scope of nursing practice but requiring a physician's order for the nurse to implement

j. any treatment, based upon clinical judgment and knowledge, that a nurse performs to enhance client outcomes

k. the desired result from nursing care expressed in terms of measurable client behaviors

Copyright © 2004, Elsevier Science (USA). All Rights Reserved.

l. preparation for moving a client from one level of care to another within or outside the current health care agency

m. a multidisciplinary plan that projects the expected course of the client's progress over the hospital stay

n. a guide for health care that identifies client problems in need of nursing care, predicts outcomes sensitive to nursing care, and lists interventions that should result in the expected outcomes

o. a standardized language for measuring the effects of nursing care using indicators sensitive to nursing intervention

p. suggests that the expectation for resolution of the nursing diagnosis will take place in small measurable steps but may take a few weeks or months

TRUE OR FALSE

17. ____ Planning occurs only at the beginning of the nurse-client relationship.

18. ____ A nursing care plan for clients who are undergoing a hysterectomy is sufficient for all hysterectomy clients.

19. ____ The nursing care plan does not include interventions performed by other team members, such as the dietitian.

20. ____ Planning includes projecting the desired outcomes of the care.

21. ____ Priorities are always based on physiological needs first.

22. ____ Because needs are often interrelated, several problems may be grouped together as a priority.

23. ____ To use the Nursing Outcomes Classification system, the nurse must choose which measurement parameters are needed in a given client situation.

24. ____ Nursing interventions are clarified by indicating who, what, when, how, and why.

25. ____ Nursing practice that consistently upholds standards of care is important in achieving positive client outcomes.

26. ____ If client outcomes are not achieved, only the nursing interventions are revised.

27. ____ Nurses can often determine a client's level of satisfaction with care by asking the opinions of other nurses assigned to that client.

28. ____ Formulating measurable and realistic client outcomes is a factor that facilitates attainment of those outcomes.

29. ____ Inadequate information about a client's disease, treatment, or care is a barrier that impedes attainment of expected outcomes.

30. ____ A nurse using a clinical pathway in the care of an assigned client would document the reasons for any variances in the client's medical record.

FILL-IN-THE-BLANKS

31. The frequency of planning during a client's span of care depends on how often the client's condition _____.

32. Basic survival needs take first priority when your client has a threat to _____ _____.

33. Nursing diagnoses are documented in the health care record in the _____ care plan or the _____ care plan.

34. Through the development of expected outcomes, nurses can be held _____ for the results of nursing care.

35. In planning nursing care you should choose outcomes that are _____ to nursing care.

36. The Nursing Outcomes Classification system uses a _____- or _____-point scale to measure outcomes, thus allowing for variable client outcomes.

37. A standardized language provides a common language for _____.

38. If a client has begun to achieve expected outcomes, but has not yet fully met them, the nurse would consider that the goals for this client have been _____ met.

39. A nurse whose evaluation shows that a client has fully met the expected outcomes for a nursing diagnosis would determine that the nursing diagnosis should be _____.

40. A factor that impedes the ability of a client to meet an expected outcome is considered to be a _____.

41. Criteria used to measure competent practice of the ANA standards of care are called _____.

Copyright © 2004, Elsevier Science (USA). All Rights Reserved.

TEST YOURSELF

42. All of the following interventions are missing some of the five elements of who, what, when, how, and why. Select the one you think would be the most consistently carried out across all three shifts.
    1. Turn q2h
    2. Turn on even hours, side to back to side
    3. Turn as needed to prevent decubiti
    4. Instruct nursing assistant to turn client

43. You refer a client to AIDS Services (a local volunteer agency) for assistance in obtaining medication. Which domain of interventions (NIC) have you used?
    1. Physiological
    2. Behavioral
    3. Safety
    4. Health systems

44. Your client needs to learn to give an injection to himself on a weekly basis. Which of the following would be the most measurable client outcome?
    1. Understands the mechanics of the injection technique
    2. Demonstrates the correct injection technique before discharge
    3. Develops a procedure for injection suitable to his lifestyle
    4. Knows how to give his own injection

45. A client has a fractured ankle. He is learning to walk on crutches. Which of the following outcomes best reflects the client's long-term goal?
    1. Safely demonstrates stair climbing with crutches
    2. Can walk the length of the corridor correctly using a three-point gait
    3. Can use crutches independently at discharge
    4. Bears weight on ankle without pain

46. Which of the following nursing activities most clearly reflects a nurse-initiated intervention?
    1. Safely administers intravenous gentamicin (Garamycin)
    2. Establishes schedule for the administration of medication
    3. Observes for side effects of medication
    4. Teaches client to self-administer medication after discharge

47. Which of the following would be the most significant disadvantage of a computerized nursing care plan?
    1. Difficult care plan development and revision
    2. Low rating for readability
    3. Lack of individualization
    4. Lack of clarity of the terms used in planning

48. Select the statement that reflects an advantage to the NIC system for documentation of interventions.
    1. Each intervention is specific for a NANDA diagnosis.
    2. NIC provides ease of documentation of individualized care.
    3. NIC provides the specific details of the activities used for each client.
    4. NIC provides a short notation that implies the same set of activities to all who use the system.

49. Select the statement that best exemplifies the purpose of case management. It seeks to:
    1. ensure quality care in a health care system focused on cost control.
    2. expand the hospital's control beyond the acute care experience.
    3. increase the number of roles for professional nurses in acute care.
    4. ensure that clients get access to all possible services.

50. Which of the following statements best describes a clinical pathway?
    1. Describes the specifics of nursing care in measurable terms
    2. Is a multidisciplinary plan with criteria for daily progress of a client with a particular diagnosis
    3. Is a plan of care for an individual client
    4. Predicts the course of a client's illness based on the identification of that client's individual risk factors

51. There are multiple methods of documenting a nursing care plan (NCP). Which of the following is essential?
    1. Using a form developed for the agency for documentation of the NCP
    2. Using columns for expected outcomes, interventions, and resolution of the problem
    3. Documenting the elements of diagnosis, expected outcomes, and interventions
    4. Having the plan on a separate form from the documentation of care

52. A nurse who is facilitating a client's attainment of expected outcomes would:
    1. have a vague idea of the client's plan of care.
    2. assess the client thoroughly and accurately.
    3. not be overly concerned with revising the plan of care.
    4. consult with the family, but not the client, about expected outcomes.

Copyright © 2004, Elsevier Science (USA). All Rights Reserved.

53. The nurse would determine that a case management approach was most effective if the client:
    1. is approved by the insurance company to remain in the hospital an extra day or two.
    2. achieved a satisfactory clinical outcome and did not require rehospitalization.
    3. received every type of service available.
    4. incurred the least cost even if the outcome was less than desireable.

Copyright © 2004, Elsevier Science (USA). All Rights Reserved.

Documenting Care

PURPOSE

This chapter explains the purpose, principles, and methods of documenting client care. It differentiates among the various charting formats and describes the usefulness of various types of flow sheets.

MATCHING

1. ____ admit note/admission note

2. ____ APIE charting

3. ____ charting by exception

4. ____ clinical pathways (care maps)/critical pathways

5. ____ computer-based records

6. ____ discharge note

7. ____ documentation

8. ____ flow sheet

9. ____ focus charting

10. ____ interval or progress note

11. ____ narrative charting

12. ____ PIE charting

13. ____ problem-oriented medical records

14. ____ SOAP charting

15. ____ source-oriented medical records

16. ____ transfer note

   a. nursing note that reflects the circumstances surrounding the release of a client from a facility

   b. a method of charting that addresses client problems or needs and includes a column that summarizes the focus of the entry

   c. a method of charting that provides information in the form of statements that describe events surrounding client care

   d. the first nurse's note acknowledging the arrival of a new client

   e. a type of medical record with separate divisions according to health discipline (e.g., medicine, nursing, laboratory, respiratory care)

   f. the acronym that stands for assessment, problem identification, interventions, and evaluation

   g. the acronym that stands for problem identification, interventions, and evaluation

   h. a form of documentation originally designed to organize information according to identified client problems, with all members of the health team documenting information sequentially

   i. recording of information relevant to assessment, planning, implementation, and evaluation (client response) as a legal record that is permanent and retrievable for future purposes

   j. forms used to document data that can be more easily followed in graphic or tabular form

   k. provides documentation in progress notes only if data are significant or abnormal

   l. nursing notes entered at various times during a shift that reflect any aspect of change in client condition, or anything affecting the client such as tests, STAT or prn medications, and procedures

   m. nursing note that reflects the movement of a client from one unit to another within the agency or to another agency

   n. a format of charting used to record progress notes with problem-focused charting; it includes subjective data, objective data, assessment, and plan

   o. used in many health care settings to facilitate delivery of patient care and support date analysis necessary for strategic planning

   p. may be recorded using an interdisciplinary approach or organized by health care discipline

Copyright © 2004, Elsevier Science (USA). All Rights Reserved.

TRUE OR FALSE

17. ____ Client outcomes serve as the measure of quality and are monitored through complete and accurate documentation.

18. ____ Agencies do not chart errors in clients' charts to avoid being sued.

19. ____ Medical abbreviations are used consistently throughout the medical/nursing community.

20. ____ Charting should be done in complete sentences, using as much description of the situation as possible.

21. ____ You are responsible for charting how your client responds to your teaching, and whether the client and/or family can return-demonstrate a skill such as wound care or explain the instructions in their own words.

22. ____ Narrative charting is unstructured, providing you with flexibility in determining how information is recorded.

23. ____ The use of computer systems for documentation has raised concerns over confidentiality and security of client information.

FILL-IN-THE-BLANKS

24. The primary purpose of _____ of a client's care is _____ among health team members thus promoting continuity of care among departments, throughout 24 hours of care, and during the entire hospital stay.

25. Quality assurance focuses on providing care according to established_____.

26. _____ is the choice of color for charting, unless an agency has a different policy.

27. When you chart you do not include the_____ name or the word *client* or *patient*.

28. Copying a chart usually requires written consent by the_____ or responsible party.

29. Upon admission to a facility, documentation of the client's _____ to the facility should be made.

30. Nursing notes should state_____ rather than opinion.

EXERCISING YOUR CLINICAL JUDGMENT

31. You admitted Ms. Peters, the client mentioned at the beginning of the textbook chapter, to your hospital unit. You charted: *68-yr-old female admitted to room 268A via stretcher from ER with dx FX L h P 92, BP142/89, T 98. C/o pain to L hip from mid-thigh to greater trochanter area, marked bruising noted in same area.* The agency where you work is using which type of charting format?
    1. Narrative
    2. Focus
    3. APIE
    4. Charting by exception

32. You charted the following nursing note in black ink: *12:00 ate lunch; 7:30 AM prn medication given for pain; 1:00 transferred to X-ray via a stretcher, accompanied by aide.* What is incorrect about this entry?
    1. The prn medication should not have been recorded.
    2. The recording of the information is not done sequentially.
    3. Black ink is not the ink of choice for most institutions.
    4. The charting should have included the client's name.

33. Ms. Peters, the elderly client from the chapter's case study, has been on your unit for several days. You chart the following: *Dr. Warren visited with orders to d/c current meds. Neighbor notified and on the way. Home Health Nurse notified of discharge and arrangement for first visit made. PT visited concerning walker and reinforced proper use.* This is an example of which type of nursing note?
    1. Progress
    2. Interval
    3. Discharge
    4. Assessment

Copyright © 2004, Elsevier Science (USA). All Rights Reserved.

TEST YOURSELF

34. Your client has his dressing changed every 4 hours. You forgot to chart the morning dressing change. You remembered the omission when you began to document your client's afternoon dressing change. The client's morning dressing had no drainage on it and the wound was healing without any problems. How would you handle this situation?
    1. Chart the morning results with your afternoon charting.
    2. Call the physician and report you did not chart the dressing change the client's chart.
    3. Add the information as an addendum to the afternoon charting.
    4. Do nothing; because the dressing is changed frequently, it is not necessary to add the morning dressing change to the client's chart.

35. You are about to chart and notice that the previous charting was not signed. How should you chart?
    1. Sign the previous nurse's charting and then do your charting and sign it.
    2. Have the head nurse sign the previous nurse's charting and then do your own.
    3. No is action necessary; do only your own charting.
    4. Do not sign for the previous nurse; report it to the head nurse and chart and sign your own charting.

36. You charted the following nursing note regarding your client's current condition: *Awake, alert and oriented x3. Skin warm and dry. IV D_5W infusing in R lower arm at 100cc/h with 450 TBA. Site without redness or edema. Reports pain in L hip. States pain is 8 on scale of 1–10. Tylox tabs ii given PO.* Which type of nursing note is this?
    1. Admit note
    2. Change-of-shift note
    3. Assessment note
    4. Interval note

37. You chart a progress note on your client's condition using the same problem list as the client's other health care providers used. What type of medical record is your facility using?
    1. Source-oriented
    2. Problem-oriented
    3. Critical pathways
    4. Narrative

38. Which type of charting addresses client problems or needs and includes a column that summarizes the focus of the entry?
    1. Focus
    2. SOAP
    3. Narrative
    4. PIE

Copyright © 2004, Elsevier Science (USA). All Rights Reserved.

12

The Nurse-Client Relationship

PURPOSE

This chapter will orient you to beginning theories, principles, and techniques of therapeutic communication related to the nurse-client interaction.

MATCHING

1. ____ acting-out behaviors
2. ____ active listening
3. ____ attending behaviors
4. ____ body language
5. ____ context
6. ____ decoder (receiver)
7. ____ empathy
8. ____ encoder (sender)
9. ____ feedback
10. ____ language
11. ____ message
12. ____ nonverbal communication
13. ____ paralanguage
14. ____ personal space
15. ____ sensory channel
16. ____ therapeutic rapport
17. ____ therapeutic relationship
18. ____ unconditional positive regard
19. ____ verbal communication

a. a helping relationship

b. a special bond that exists between a nurse and a client who have established a sense of trust and a

mutual understanding of what will occur in their relationship

c. inappropriate or unexpected client behaviors that communicate the client's true or subconscious feelings and concerns

d. person who initiates a transaction to exchange information, convey thoughts and feelings, or engage another person

e. the content a sender wishes to transmit to another person (the receiver) in the process of communication

f. the means by which a message is sent

g. a person to whom a message is aimed

h. the condition under which a communication occurs

i. the process by which effectiveness of communication is determined

j. involves the use of words to convey messages

k. a set of words that have meanings that are comprehensible within a group

l. a set of behaviors that convey messages either without words or by supplementing verbal communication

m. refers to nonverbal communication behaviors that are accomplished by the movement of our bodies or body parts, by the presentation of ourselves to the world, and by the use of our personal space

n. refers to nonverbal components of spoken language

o. a private zone or "bubble" around our body that we believe is an extension of ourselves

p. shows that you are paying attention and listening to what the client is saying

Copyright © 2004, Elsevier Science (USA). All Rights Reserved.

q. term coined by psychologist Carl Rogers; describes respect for the client that is not dependent on the client's behavior

r. the accurate perception of the client's feelings

s. understanding not only the words spoken but also the feeling and intent behind the message

TRUE OR FALSE

20. ____ A therapeutic relationship is personal, client-focused, and aimed at realizing mutually determined goals.

21. ____ Peplau, a nurse theorist, believed that the nurse is a human being who is vulnerable to stereotypes, labels, and generalizations.

22. ____ Nonverbal communication includes body posture.

23. ____ Generally speaking, a person's personal space is similar for most cultures.

24. ____ A rule of thumb is to ask permission before touching a client.

25. ____ According to Tannen's theories, women speak to connect and men speak to preserve status and independence.

26. ____ To encourage a formulation of a plan of action, you should consider what might be the best thing to do in a future situation.

27. ____ Summarizing can help bring closure in the termination phase of a therapeutic relationship.

FILL-IN-THE-BLANKS

28. Confidentiality is an _____ obligation to share a client's health care information only with other persons who have a _____ need to know his or her health status.

29. _____ feedback affirms your efforts to communicate by rewarding and reinforcing successful communication.

30. Personal appearance, conscious and unconscious changes in facial expressions, body posture and gestures, and the distances maintained from others are examples of common _____ _____ behaviors.

31. You can help the client who is experiencing a misperception of reality by using a technique called _____ _____.

32. If you are using therapeutic techniques correctly, your client will be doing most of the _____ as you listen and guide the interaction.

33. Many people (nurses and clients) are uncomfortable with _____ and will talk continuously about nothing in particular just to avoid it.

34. _____ listening is a means of "being with" the client and indicating acceptance and agreement by using verbal and nonverbal cues.

EXERCISING YOUR CLINICAL JUDGMENT

35. You say to Mr. Lewis, the client from the chapter's case study, "Why are you afraid of a simple surgery?" This is an example of which type of nontherapeutic technique?
   1. Requesting an explanation
   2. Probing
   3. Challenging
   4. Testing

36. You say to Mr. Lewis, "Would you mind explaining more about what you mean so I can be more helpful?" You are using which therapeutic communication technique?
   1. Offering self
   2. Focusing
   3. Asking for clarification
   4. Reflecting

37. You say to your Mr. Lewis, "Tell me what I can cover next about your surgery." This is an example of which therapeutic communication technique?
   1. Providing broad openings
   2. Focusing
   3. Summarizing
   4. Reflecting

TEST YOURSELF

38. "I don't know the answer right now. But I will find out and let you know in an about hour." This is an example of being honest with the client, which is an essential step in:
   1. developing a trusting relationship with the client.
   2. developing a friendship with the client.
   3. helping the client with termination issues.
   4. believing that you are a competent nurse.

Copyright © 2004, Elsevier Science (USA). All Rights Reserved.

39. During which phase of the nurse-client relationship do you complete nursing interventions that address expected nursing outcomes?
    1. Working phase
    2. Termination phase
    3. Orientation phase
    4. Therapeutic phase

40. "Hmm, I believe you are right," is an example of which type of paralanguage?
    1. Rate
    2. Pitch
    3. Quality
    4. Pause

41. You say to your adult client, "I have 30 minutes available to talk with you at 10 AM today." This is an example of which therapeutic communication technique?
    1. Offering self
    2. Presenting reality
    3. Focusing
    4. Testing

42. You say to your client who is 3 years old, "Do you want your Baby Lisa? Is she your doll?" Which therapeutic communication techniques are you using?
    1. Focusing
    2. Placing events in sequence
    3. Providing broad openings
    4. Seeking consensual validation

Copyright © 2004, Elsevier Science (USA). All Rights Reserved.

13

Client Teaching

PURPOSE

This chapter introduces you to the key concepts that you must understand to provide effective client teaching. It introduces teaching-learning theory and processes, and guides you to use the nursing process effectively in meeting clients' learning needs.

MATCHING

1. ____ learning objective

2. ____ teaching plan

3. ____ psychomotor learning domain

4. ____ teaching

5. ____ learning

6. ____ cognitive learning domain

7. ____ affective learning domain

8. ____ learning contract

   a. includes physical and motor skills, such as giving injections

   b. much like any business contract; each party, nurse and client, agrees to contribute certain things to the agreement

   c. considered the "thinking" domain and includes acquiring knowledge, comprehending, and using critical thinking skills

   d. a set of planned activities performed to impact knowledge, behavior, or skill

   e. includes ethics, principles, and reasoning that determine and guide moral or "right" behavior

   f. acquisition of knowledge, behavior, or skill through experience, practice, study, or instruction.

   g. describes the intended results of learning rather than the process of instruction

   h. an organized, individualized written presentation of what the client must learn and how the instructions and information needed will be provided

TRUE OR FALSE

9. ____ JCAHO, the Joint Commission on Accreditation of Healthcare Organizations, has included client education within their nursing standard since 1993.

10. ____ Client education is a factor in quality control in that it ensures that clients have the knowledge they need to provide self-care.

11. ____ The client must reach the synthesis level of learning about his of her health care problem to be successful.

12. ____ In the United States, literacy is not a concern for those who provide client education.

13. ____ A child's imagination may create greater fear than the truth, told directly and simply.

14. ____ For the adult learner you should assume that the learner has some knowledge you can use to build on to enhance education.

15. ____ In a hospital setting, the best method of teaching is verbally providing information in a one-on-one situation with the client.

16. ____ It is safe to assume all clients want to learn about their health problems.

17. ____ *Deficit knowledge* is the only nursing diagnosis used for client learning needs.

18. ____ Teaching from the simple to the complex is a principle of teaching.

19. ____ Writing specific measurable objectives helps to clarify your teaching plans.

FILL-IN-THE-BLANKS

20. The advantage of _____ instruction is pacing and customizing to meet an individual client's needs.

21. The advantage of _____ instruction is economy of teaching time and sharing of experiences.

Copyright © 2004, Elsevier Science (USA). All Rights Reserved.

43

22. The advantage of _____ materials is they are affordable and can be used to teach or reinforce a learning experience.

23. Repetition is used to _____ _____.

24. Discussion allows the learner to be an _____ _____ in learning.

25. Evaluation has two types of goals. Assessing the client's ability to repeat the information is a _____-_____ goal.

26. Assessing for a change in lifestyle at a 3-month follow-up is a _____-_____ goal.

EXERCISING YOUR CLINICAL JUDGMENT

27. Mrs. Avery, the client from the case study, is going to go home on a new medication to control her diabetes (insulin). Based on the axiom that adult learners learn best when there is a need to know, which of the following would you emphasize?
    1. How the medication works in the body
    2. The need to memorize all side effects
    3. The importance of maintaining the prescribed dose schedule
    4. The possible complications of diabetes

28. Which of the following is most likely true of Mrs. Avery as an adult learner?
    1. Prefers the nurse to identify what knowledge is needed
    2. Is bored with being shown how to perform a skill
    3. Likes to know why knowledge is needed
    4. Likes role playing as a method of learning

29. Mrs. Avery indicates she has the greatest motivation to learn when she does which of the following?
    1. Asks questions about giving herself insulin.
    2. Thanks the nurse and says she will read the information provided
    3. Talks about the difficulties of giving herself insulin
    4. Tells the nurse to talk to her granddaughter about the insulin injections

TEST YOURSELF

30. Your client has just been admitted with an asthma attack. This is the third admission in 6 months and the client is highly anxious. You suspect the client does not fully understand the preventive measures recommended by the physician. You would:
    1. review the measures while the client is waiting for the medications to take effect.
    2. gather limited information at this time and postpone teaching.
    3. give the client written information to be read later.
    4. use the opportunity to emphasize the importance of prevention.

31. The physician has recommended that your client follow a low-fat diet and wants you to introduce the topic to the client. Knowing you should teach from the simple to the complex you would start with the topic of:
    1. a general list of foods to avoid.
    2. pathophysiology of the formation of fatty plaque in arteries.
    3. planning menus.
    4. maintaining a diet that is less than 30% fat based on grams of fat in common foods.

32. Early discharge for hospitalized clients has changed client teaching by:
    1. increasing the client's need for information.
    2. shifting the responsibility for teaching from the hospital nurse to the home health nurse.
    3. reducing the need for teaching because complications are reduced.
    4. allowing hospital nurses to focus only on acute physical needs.

33. Quality care is improved when:
    1. the client and family are active participants in restoring health.
    2. clients do what they are told without asking questions.
    3. the physician is in control of all decision making.
    4. clients have absolute faith in health care providers.

34. Which behavior represents the complex overt response level of psychomotor learning?
    1. Performs the skill precisely following the steps as taught
    2. Performs the skill correctly while visiting with a friend
    3. Modifies the skill to meet lifestyle needs
    4. Creates a new way of performing the skill

Copyright © 2004, Elsevier Science (USA). All Rights Reserved.

35. Your client is a shy 7-year-old. She is learning to use an asthma inhaler. Her asthma attacks occur no more frequently than once a week. Her mother has received permission from the school for the child to have the inhaler with her in the classroom, but the child says she cannot use it in front of her friends. Which teaching activity would you select?
    1. Telling her that her friends won't care
    2. Role-play asking the teacher if she can be excused from the room to use her inhaler
    3. Getting the prescription changed to a tablet taken four times a day
    4. Telling her mother that she has to do it whether she likes it or not

36. Your client is having surgery and expects to be in the hospital for 4 days. The postoperative care will involve complex wound care after discharge. The best time to start the teaching is:
    1. preoperatively.
    2. on the first day after surgery.
    3. on the day of discharge.
    4. after the client is at home.

37. Select the client who would most likely need repetition to ensure learning.
    1. A 90-year-old using insulin injections for the first time
    2. A 20-year-old who needs to take a prescription for 10 days for a urinary tract infection
    3. A person with long-standing asthma who has a prescription for a different inhaler
    4. A surgical client being discharged; wound is healing without complications and the sutures have been removed

38. You have planned to do a client's wound care at 10 AM. Your schedule is busy and you know the client will probably be discharged tomorrow. When you enter the room, you find that the client's son has just arrived from out of state. You would:
    1. know that psychosocial needs are important and delay the wound care.
    2. ask the son to leave the room and hurriedly do the wound care without teaching.
    3. ask the client if the son can stay and include him in the teaching.
    4. tell the son he will have to come back later.

Copyright © 2004, Elsevier Science (USA). All Rights Reserved.

Managing Client Care

PURPOSE

This chapter introduces you to nursing management and the roles of a nurse–manager at different levels in an organization. It describes how these roles involve managing quality, budgets, people, change, and risk.

MATCHING

1. ____ accountability

2. ____ authority

3. ____ change-of-shift report

4. ____ delegation

5. ____ leadership

6. ____ management

7. ____ nurse–manager

8. ____ primary nursing

9. ____ quality assurance

10. ____ responsibility

11. ____ risk management

12. ____ team nursing

a. being held answerable for personal actions or the actions of others

b. the obligation to provide an accounting or rationale for personal actions or the actions of others

c. a nurse responsible for managing the operation and expenses of a health care organization that employs nurses as the means to produce health

d. the process of identifying, evaluating, and reducing or financing the cost of predictable losses

e. the ability or legitimate power to make decisions, implement strategies, and elicit work from others

f. involves assigning responsibility for certain tasks to other people, thereby allowing the manager to concentrate on organizational goals and productivity

g. involves showing others the way, directing others in a course of action, going before others, or going with and inspiring others

h. the implementation of strategies that promote effective and efficient use of resources to achieve organizational goals

i. refers to the process of achieving an optimal degree of excellence in the services rendered to every client

j. a combination of nursing personnel who work together and share responsibility for the care of a group of clients

k. enhances comprehensive care by assigning each client to a nurse at the bedside who is responsible for the client's care over a 24-hour period

l. an oral report given by an off-going nurse to an on-coming nurse who will assume responsibility for the care of a client.

TRUE OR FALSE

13. ____ Nurse–managers have become consensus builders who facilitate client care rather than acting as control systems.

14. ____ A nurse–manager who wanted to hire a new nurse could use information gained as part of fiscal management to justify the need.

15. ____ The overall definition of the business of health care for each institution is written in the form of a policy.

16. ____ A mission statement is used to identify institutional goals.

17. ____ Organizational goals are translated into specific objectives to guide the day-to-day operation of work units.

18. ____ Cost containment remains a major goal in health care today and affects all health care practitioners.

 Copyright © 2004, Elsevier Science (USA). All Rights Reserved.

19. ____ An institution must be accredited by the JCAHO to be certified or licensed, or to receive reimbursement for services.

20. ____ A nurse who is verifying information for properly submitting a vacation request form would consult the nursing procedure manual.

FILL-IN-THE-BLANKS

21. A female nurse orientee who requests that the designated mentor nurse observe her while she performs a wound irrigation is engaged in the _____ audit method.

22. An assumption of a continuous quality improvement program is that quality can always be _____.

23. Regardless of whether the setting is a home care agency or a hospital, the goal of a nurse manager is to promote_____.

24. Because the position of a nurse–manager involves inspiring others to work, all nurse–managers should be _____.

25. An _____ is defined as a social system deliberately established to carry out some defining purpose.

26. Most organizations create a diagram called an _____ _____ that depicts the hierarchical arrangement of its managers.

27. Managing _____ means accentuating positive outcomes as well as avoiding negative outcomes.

28. Nurse–managers evaluate how well policies and procedures facilitate the attainment of goals by measuring _____.

29. _____ and _____ are rules and outlined processes that define the steps taken to meet objectives.

30. Nurse–managers strive to ensure the highest quality care at the lowest possible _____.

EXERCISING YOUR CLINICAL JUDGMENT

Kristen Williams is a nurse–manager on a 40-bed surgical unit in a local hospital. She arrived at work at 7 AM and is developing her plan for the day after reviewing her scheduled appointments and meetings. She must attend a 9 AM meeting of the Policy and Procedure Committee, followed by a budget meeting at 10 AM. In the afternoon she has a staff meeting planned to explore with staff how they can achieve more timely client discharges on the unit before new admissions arrive from the postanesthesia care unit. As she gathers the materials needed for the morning meetings, she realizes that in her role today she will be managing quality, people, budget, and change. She glances at her watch and determines that she has plenty of time to talk to the charge nurse and nursing staff about concerns on the unit before her planned schedule begins.

31. As Kristen enters the nurses' station, the charge nurse reports that there has been a sick call already for the evening shift. Which of the following actions would represent the best use of Kristen's time and skills and those of other staff?
    1. Delegate to the charge nurse the responsibility for calling part-time off-duty nurses to see if they can work
    2. Call the vice president for nursing to complain about how short-staffed the unit always is
    3. Make a mental note to bring this problem up at the budget meeting and try to use it to demand more staff
    4. Tell the staff at 3 PM that they will have to work short and "make do."

32. At the Policy and Procedure Committee meeting, the first item on the agenda is a review of the effectiveness of a new policy and procedure for blood transfusion intended to reduce turn-around time from receipt of an order in the blood bank to the start time for infusion into the client. The committee determines that based on data available, 20 minutes have been eliminated in the process. The new policy and procedure are determined to be effective in improving which of the following?
    1. Communication
    2. Quality
    3. Cost
    4. Goals

33. At the budget meeting, Kristen must determine projected revenue from her nursing unit for the coming year. She would use concepts related to which of the following in order to complete this work?
    1. Negotiation
    2. Lobbying
    3. Forecasting
    4. Staffing

TEST YOURSELF

34. Which of the following members of the hospital staff would not be part of a multidisciplinary team working with a client?
    1. Social worker
    2. Billing clerk
    3. Pastoral care provider
    4. Client's family

Copyright © 2004, Elsevier Science (USA). All Rights Reserved.

35. Which of the following activities undertaken as part of a planned change correlates with the analysis phase of the nursing process?
    1. Identify the need for change
    2. Identify potential action plans
    3. Identify the potential cause of a problem
    4. Incorporate new behaviors into structures or processes

36. Which of the following time management tips would be least useful and productive for a nurse–manager?
    1. Write down identified tasks, obligations, and activities
    2. Work on the most important task first
    3. Do not accept assignments that you are not capable of completing
    4. Adopt a strategy of needing to be perfect

37. The nurse–managers of an institution are meeting to determine how well they are complying with regulations of the Joint Commission on Accreditation of Healthcare Organizations. The group is motivated to be in compliance because this is necessary for:
    1. praise from the chief executive officer.
    2. national recognition.
    3. accreditation.
    4. high profit margins.

38. A client expresses satisfaction with the nursing care received on the clinical unit, and completes a patient satisfaction survey describing it as caring, thoughtful, and respectful. The nurse–manager documents this anecdote from the client, knowing that this information is an example of which of the following?
    1. Quality indicator
    2. Internal standard
    3. External standard
    4. Compliance with federal regulation

39. The nurse who is practicing nursing within the standards of a specialty nursing organization knows that these standards most often are derived from those of which of the following?
    1. Employer
    2. Joint Commission on Accreditation of Healthcare Organizations
    3. Department of Health and Human Services
    4. American Nurses Association

40. A nurse working on the cardiac telemetry unit has a set of standing physician's orders for treating chest pain. The nurse implementing these orders is working with which of the following?
    1. Policy
    2. Procedure
    3. Protocol
    4. Parameter

Copyright © 2004, Elsevier Science (USA). All Rights Reserved.

15

Nursing Research

PURPOSE

The purpose of this chapter is to provide introductory information about nursing research and its methodology to assist you in reading research studies.

MATCHING

1. ____ abstract

2. ____ data

3. ____ data collection

4. ____ dependent variable

5. ____ experimental research

6. ____ hypothesis

7. ____ independent variable

8. ____ informed consent

9. ____ institutional review board

10. ____ instruments

11. ____ nonexperimental research

12. ____ operational definition

13. ____ qualitative research

14. ____ quantitative research

15. ____ quasi-experimental research

16. ____ research design

17. ____ research problem

18. ____ sampling

19. ____ theoretical framework

a. a short summary that contains brief information about the purpose of the study, the number of subjects, methodology used to select subjects, the type of study being conducted, and the major results from the study

b. the process by which the researcher acquires subjects and collects the information necessary to answer the research question

c. a type of research study in which the researcher manipulates a treatment or intervention, randomly assigns subjects to either a control or experimental group, and has control over the research situation

d. a tentative prediction of the relationship between two or more variables being studied

e. the variable in a research design that may show variation, but the variation is expected to remain constant in the study, although it influences or even causes change in another variable

f. the tools a researcher uses to conduct a study

g. the variable in a research design that is hypothesized to change with the treatment (i.e., has been caused by an independent variable)

h. used to designate the information the researcher is interested in collecting

i. a type of study in which the researcher collects data without the introduction of a treatment or intervention

j. a type of study that uses ideas that are analyzed as words

k. a type of study in which the researcher manipulates a treatment or intervention, but is unable to randomize subjects into groups or lacks a control group

l. a committee whose duties include ensuring that the proposed research meets the federal requirements for ethical research; the federal government mandates the committee if the institution is receiving federal funds for research

m. means that the subjects have been provided with sufficient information regarding the research to

Copyright © 2004, Elsevier Science (USA). All Rights Reserved.

enable them to consent voluntarily to participate or decline to participate.

n. a type of study that uses variables that are analyzed as numbers

o. the meaning of the concept precisely as it is being used in the study, defined in a manner that specifies how the concepts will be measured

p. a researcher's strategy for testing a hypothesis

q. the process of collecting data from a portion of the group being studied

r. an observation, situation, occurrence, or even a hunch that an investigator chooses to research

s. a logical but abstract structure that suggests the relationship among the variables for a research study

TRUE OR FALSE

20. ____ One of the ANA priorities for nursing research is to analyze home health care services and data on elders at home and in long-term care facilities.

21. ____ One of the priorities for the National Center for Nursing Research is to test interventions for coping with chronic illness.

22. ____ Informed consent for research includes a clear statement that the subject is free to discontinue participation at any time the subject wishes.

23. ____ In the absence of a requirement for institutional review, researchers are free to skip some ethical guidelines.

24. ____ Research should not be performed on human subjects unless there is a clear possibility of benefit to society or individuals.

25. ____ When a research study shows a good correlation between two variables, causation can be inferred.

26. ____ Reading an abstract is sufficient to evaluate a study.

27. ____ The results of a study are a factual presentation of what is found.

28. ____ In the discussion that follows the results, the researcher tells what the findings mean in his or her opinion.

29. ____ Not all problems are amenable to research methods.

30. ____ The *Index Medicus* does not contain nursing journals.

31. ____ As a user of research, the operational definition can help you know if the information applies in a specific client situation.

32. ____ A research study is not worthwhile unless it proves the hypothesis.

33. ____ Research begins with a problem or a question that arises in the clinical practice setting.

34. ____ When you are reading a research study, always ask, "What else could have caused this effect?"

35. ____ The goal of using research findings is to improve the quality of care in the clinical setting.

FILL-IN-THE-BLANKS

36. _____ _____ is the method used to develop or search for knowledge about issues important to nurses and nursing practice.

37. _____ _____ was the first nurse researcher.

38. Because nursing research often involves _____ _____, ethical standards are especially important.

39. A _____ _____ is a type of research that involves the detailed investigation of an individual, group, or institution to understand which variables are important to the subjects—history, care, or development.

40. The concepts under investigation in a study are called _____.

41. In a _____ (random, nonrandom) sample each member of the population has an equal chance of being selected as part of the sample.

42. In qualitative research the data are analyzed by _____ of large volumes of narrative data into categories that can be identified as the concepts present in the situation.

43. Controlling _____ variables controls research bias.

44. When you ask if the passage of time has affected the results, you are asking a question about the validity classification of _____.

45. _____ refers to whether it makes good sense to attempt an innovation in your practice situation.

Copyright © 2004, Elsevier Science (USA). All Rights Reserved.

TEST YOURSELF

46. Select the statement that is true about the case study method of research.
    1. Case studies increase knowledge of clients with similar conditions.
    2. Case studies are not a valid method of research.
    3. Case studies focus on the psychosocial needs of clients.
    4. Case studies rule out the need to consider multiple variables.

47. Before you use the findings of a research study to make decisions in the clinical setting, you should make which of the following determinations?
    1. Whether the elements of the situation are precisely like those of the study
    2. Whether you have the qualifications to make decisions using research
    3. Whether your hospital is a research hospital
    4. Whether the elements of the situation are sufficiently similar to the conditions of study to make it likely that the intervention will work in this situation

48. Which of the following items would be consistent with one of the ANA priorities for nursing research?
    1. Finding a cure for AIDS
    2. Testing lifestyle management strategies for preventing AIDS
    3. Developing a vaccine against AIDS
    4. Describing the mutation mechanisms of the HIV virus

49. Select the most important criterion for deciding if a problem is worth studying.
    1. The solution can be expected to improve the quality of life for a number of clients.
    2. The solution to the problem will make the researcher famous.
    3. The problem is unusual and therefore interesting to study.
    4. Enough is known about the problem to make a solution feasible.

50. A nurse wants to study a technique for reducing infection rates in premature infants. Select the behavior that would be within ethical guidelines for research.
    1. Not informing the parents of the control group because nothing will change for their child
    2. Not informing the parents of the experimental group because their participation is not necessary
    3. Selecting the babies with greater weights for the experimental group to prevent causing harm
    4. Fully informing and seeking consent from parents of all infants

51. At which of the following times is the review of a research protocol by an institutional review board required?
    1. When federal support is sought to conduct the study
    2. Only when invasive procedures are used in the study
    3. Only when the subject is of a sensitive nature
    4. Only when the methods are known to cause harm

52. When considering the issue of informed consent for research, a vulnerable population is one that has which of the following characteristics?
    1. Is unable to give informed consent
    2. Is more likely to be harmed by the intervention
    3. Is at greater risk for complications
    4. Is unlikely to want to participate in the study

53. The population being studied refers to which of the following groups?
    1. Both the research subjects and the control group
    2. The group with the characteristics of the people who are selected as subjects
    3. The clients on the nursing unit where the study is being conducted
    4. Everybody living in a given geographical area

Copyright © 2004, Elsevier Science (USA). All Rights Reserved.

Infancy Through Adolescence

PURPOSE

This chapter explores concepts and principles of growth and development and factors that affect them from infancy through adolescence. It introduces you to the use of the nursing process for health maintenance and risk reduction in these client populations.

MATCHING

1. ____ attachment
2. ____ cephalocaudal
3. ____ concrete operations
4. ____ conservation
5. ____ constitutional delay of puberty
6. ____ critical periods
7. ____ development
8. ____ differentiated development
9. ____ egocentrism
10. ____ formal operations
11. ____ growth
12. ____ gynecomastia
13. ____ menarche
14. ____ nocturnal emission
15. ____ object permanence
16. ____ proximodistal
17. ____ sensory stimulation
18. ____ symbolic play

a. the physiological development of a living being and the quantitative change seen in the body

b. an absence of early signs of puberty

c. development that starts with a generalized response and progresses to a skilled specific response

d. refers to the tendency to spend so much time thinking about and focusing on your own thoughts and changes in your own body that you come to believe that others are focused on them as well

e. a progression of behavioral changes that involve the acquisition of appropriate cognitive, linguistic, and psychosocial skills

f. a benign increase in breast tissue associated with puberty

g. a discharge of semen during sleep

h. the stage of cognitive development at which children begin to project the self into other people's situations and realize that their own way of thinking isn't the only way

i. the awareness that unseen objects do not disappear; evidenced by the infant searching for an object that has been moved out of sight

j. pretend or imaginative play that enables preschool children to recreate experiences and to try out roles

k. periods of time when a person has an increased vulnerability to physical, chemical, psychological, or environmental influences

l. the time of the first menstrual period

m. a pattern of neuromuscular growth and development that starts at the head and moves toward the feet

n. a pattern of skill development that starts at the midline of the body and moves outward

Copyright © 2004, Elsevier Science (USA). All Rights Reserved.

o. the development of strong ties of affection by an infant with a significant other

p. the ability to reason abstractly

q. a child's ability to understand that changing the shape of a substance does not change its volume

r. the activation and exhilaration of the senses

TRUE OR FALSE

19. ____ Each stage of development depends on adequate completion of the previous one and forms the foundation for development of new skills.

20. ____ Jean Piaget described cognitive development as involving the increasing ability to think and reason in a logical manner.

21. ____ The list of developmental tasks is the same for all cultures.

22. ____ Crying is the primary means by which newborns make their needs and wants known.

23. ____ During parallel play, toddlers play beside, but not with, their friends.

24. ____ Socioeconomic factors, such as income, educational level, and single parenthood, influence the growth and development of children.

25. ____ The preschool years are a time of rapid weight gain for a toddler.

26. ____ It is normal for preschool children to create imaginary companions that they talk to and play with, and who become a regular part of their daily routines.

27. ____ Children between the ages of 6 and 11 have few fears, such as fear of darkness, animals, and high places.

28. ____ Children cannot be trusted to handle a gun safely, even though they have the mechanical skill and strength to fire one.

29. ____ Adolescents who are abused and neglected are at high risk for *delayed growth and development.*

30. ____ Girls are affected by a constitutional delay of puberty more often than boys are.

31. ____ Most of the cases of short stature result from underlying disease.

32. ____ The number of adolescents living with chronic illness has increased, not because the incidence of disease has changed but because more children with chronic conditions are surviving.

33. ____ Alcohol is a factor in the most common causes of deaths and injuries among adolescents.

FILL-IN-THE-BLANKS

34. A newborn's length is measured from _____ to _____.

35. Eyes begin to focus and fixate at _____ months.

36. An infant who cries when separated from parents or approached by strangers is having _____ _____.

37. Human milk is the most desirable form of milk for the first _____ months of life.

38. _____ is a genetic disorder of amino acid metabolism in which phenylalanine cannot be converted to tyrosine.

39. During the preschool years, a toddler's future body type becomes apparent. Body types include _____ (lanky build), mesomorphic (medium muscular build) and _____ (large build).

40. The vivid imagination of the _____-_____ child can turn a stuffed toy by day into a threatening monster in the dark.

41. Deaths from bicycling injuries usually result from _____ injuries and almost always are the result of _____ between bicycles and motor vehicles.

42. Children under the age of _____ should not use skateboards or in-line skates because they are not developmentally prepared to protect themselves from injury.

43. The chief developmental task of adolescence is the development of _____ versus _____.

44. Adolescents who live in poverty typically have poor nutrition, substandard housing, and limited access to _____ _____.

45. An important goal of care for hospitalized adolescents is to avoid disruption of their _____ development.

46. Adolescents with a chronic illness may engage in risk taking by failing to _____ with their treatment program.

Copyright © 2004, Elsevier Science (USA). All Rights Reserved.

EXERCISING YOUR CLINICAL JUDGMENT

Yung Hi, the 33-month-old Korean girl who was introduced in the chapter case study, has undergone orthopedic surgery to reduce a fractured femur and is in skeletal traction. She has a nursing diagnosis of *delayed growth and development* related to prescribed dependence (traction) and separation from parents at night. You are assigned to work with Yung on the evening shift, and are thus able to work with her while her mother is present, and on a one-on-one basis after the parents have gone home for the evening.

47. Which of the following age-appropriate toys would you recommend be brought to the hospital for Yung to play with during her recuperation?
    1. Mobile
    2. Rattle
    3. Toys that float in water
    4. Nontoxic crayons

48. You are trying to encourage continued physical growth during the period of recuperation. Which of the following strategies would be most useful?
    1. Try to have Yung eat the same amount of food every day.
    2. Keep foods separated from each other on the tray, and use her favorite cup at each meal.
    3. Use food as a reward for good behavior.
    4. Encourage Yung to eat every bit of food on her plate.

49. Which of the following tools would you use to assess the amount of pain that Yung is experiencing due to surgery and traction?
    1. Pain scale using words as descriptors
    2. Pain scale using numbers as descriptors
    3. Pain scale using facial expressions as descriptors
    4. A word board listing words associated with pain in Korean

50. You would plan age-appropriate care by allowing time for Yung to have a 1- to 2-hour nap each day at:
    1. 9 AM.
    2. 10 AM.
    3. 1 PM.
    4. 4 PM.

TEST YOURSELF

51. Bringing toys and games to the bedside of an immobilized child would be primarily useful interventions for which of the following nursing diagnoses?
    1. *Ineffective health maintenance*
    2. *Delayed growth and development*
    3. *Diversional activity deficit*
    4. *Health-seeking behaviors*

52. The nurse would bring rattles that make noise and vinyl or cloth books to the bedside of a client who is how old?
    1. 1 to 2 months
    2. 2 to 3 months
    3. 4 to 8 months
    4. 1 to 2 years

53. The nurse providing immunizations to children would teach the parents to report to the health care provider which of the following adverse effects of an immunization?
    1. High fever
    2. Mild discomfort at the site
    3. Rash at the site
    4. Soreness in the area

54. The home health nurse would provide parent education after noting which of the following behaviors when visiting the home of a pediatric client?
    1. All crib rails raised
    2. Mother left toddler in tub to answer door
    3. Safety handles on all cabinet doors
    4. Gate positioned at the head of the stairs

55. The nurse would avoid giving toys with small removable parts to a client younger than the age of:
    1. Six
    2. Four
    3. Three
    4. Five

56. Your client is upset because his mother left the room. She told him that she was returning in 2 hours. Fear of abandonment is a common concern for which of the following age groups?
    1. 4- to 6-year-olds
    2. Teenagers
    3. School-age children
    4. Preschoolers

57. Establishing guidelines for behavior representative of which of the following?
    1. Developing morality
    2. Discipline
    3. Limit-setting
    4. Parenting skills

58. The recommended screening for tuberculosis (TB) during childhood is at which of the following times?
    1. Twice during childhood
    2. Four times during childhood: 1, 4, 8, and 12 years old
    3. Three times during childhood: 12 to 15 months, before entering kindergarten, and at 14 to 17 years of age
    4. At entrance to school, unless otherwise indicated

Copyright © 2004, Elsevier Science (USA). All Rights Reserved.

59. Children may use symptoms such as vomiting, headaches, or abdominal pain as an excuse to say home from school because they have a fear of school. This is an example of:
    1. a phobia.
    2. school avoidance.
    3. acting-out behavior.
    4. a defense mechanism.

60. Advice you can give working parents of latchkey children is to:
    1. not leave their children unsupervised.
    2. use the community resources available to latchkey children (provide a list).
    3. encourage them have their children remain at school until they can pick them up.
    4. consider working in jobs that allow them to be at home when their children are home.

61. You are discussing preventive health issues with an adolescent client. The response you get is, "Other people may have to worry about that, but I don't have to worry about it." This is an example of which hallmark of adolescent cognitive development?
    1. Egocentrism
    2. Elitism
    3. Fantasy world
    4. Concrete thinking

62. Which of the following statements is true for constitutional delay of puberty?
    1. It affects more girls than boys, and is more likely to arise in a family in which the pubertal development of the same-sex parent was delayed.
    2. It is more likely to arise in a family in which the pubertal development of the same-sex parent was delayed.
    3. It affects more boys than girls, and is more likely to arise in a family in which the pubertal development of the same-sex parent was delayed.
    4. It affects males and females equally and is related to heredity.

63. Your adolescent client was involved in a homicide. Which of the following statements is the most accurate?
    1. Homicide is a serious public health problem in the United States, and a leading cause of deaths among young adults.
    2. Homicide-related deaths are among the top three causes of death among adolescents.
    3. Homicide deaths occur among adolescents, but are not among the primary causes of deaths among adolescents.
    4. Homicide is a serious problem because of alcohol abuse among teenagers.

64. One of the most effective ways for parents to help prevent their teenagers from becoming pregnant is to:
    1. use the "just say no" approach.
    2. buy them condoms.
    3. condone their behaviors, so they feel comfortable coming to their parents when they want advice.
    4. talk with their teenagers about sex in a nonjudgmental and informative manner.

65. Your client, a high school student, earns straight A's and is very active in school activities. She is thin and appears underdeveloped for her age. Her weight is 98 lbs. and height is 5'8". She confides in you that she feels fat. Which of the following nursing diagnoses would be most appropriate?
    1. *Ineffective health maintenance*
    2. *Ineffective individual coping*
    3. *Disturbed body image*
    4. *Delayed growth and development*

Copyright © 2004, Elsevier Science (USA). All Rights Reserved.

The Young, Middle, and Older Adult

PURPOSE

This chapter discusses key concepts related to the developmental tasks of well adults. It identifies the various factors that affect adult development. It also differentiates among the variety of diagnoses appropriate for the adult seeking knowledge or health care related to growth and development. It discusses nursing interventions to maintain health and reduce risk factors.

MATCHING

1. ____ ageism

2. ____ menopause

3. ____ middle adulthood

4. ____ midlife crisis

5. ____ older adult

6. ____ retirement

7. ____ sandwich generation

8. ____ young adulthood

   a. refers to the period from ages 20 to 35

   b. a stereotype, prejudice, or discrimination against people, particularly older adults, based on their age

   c. caught between the needs of adjacent generations; caring for ill or frail parents while handling the competing demands of children and employment

   d. any person age 65 years and older

   e. the period from ages 35 to 64

   f. a stressful life period during middle adulthood, precipitated by the review and reevaluation of one's past, including goals, priorities, and life

accomplishments, during which the person experiences inner turmoil, self-doubt, and major restructuring of personality

   g. the stage in the female climacteric, during which hormone production is reduced, the ovaries stop producing eggs, and menstruation ceases

   h. the permanent withdrawal from one's job

TRUE OR FALSE

9. ____ A person's growth and development always represent the interaction of genetic makeup and environment.

10. ____ Traditionally, biologists have divided the life span into three phases. The last phase is a decline of physical abilities after age 45.

11. ____ Erickson's theory of psychosocial development identifies the young adult stage as generativity versus stagnation.

12. ____ Regular exercise promotes appetite, mental health and balance, and reduction of stress.

13. ____ Alcohol abuse in the older adult is often very easy to determine.

14. ____ The Centers for Disease Control and Prevention (CDC) report that at least 1 in 10 deaths in North America is related to cigarette smoking.

15. ____ Stress is the most common cause of illness in our society.

16. ____ A key to wellness for the adult is appropriate screening, especially for clients in high-risk groups.

17. ____ Chronic diseases account for 70% of all deaths in the United States.

Copyright © 2004, Elsevier Science (USA). All Rights Reserved.

FILL-IN-THE-BLANKS

18. Erickson's seventh stage of psychosocial development, _____versus _____ is reached during middle adulthood.

19. Levinson conceived of development as a sequence of qualitatively distinct eras or _____, each of which has its own time and brings certain psychological challenges to the forefront of a person's life.

20. Chronic drug users are particularly susceptible to _____ _____ and are considered high-risk transmitters.

21. _____ is a stereotype, prejudice, or discrimination against people, especially older adults, based on their age.

22. Clients who are _____ experience a great deal of functional impairment, resulting in lost work time, decreased job performance, and decreased family and social functioning.

23. _____ is associated with limited access to health care, poor nutrition, substandard housing, and inadequate prenatal care.

24. The leading cause of death for adults younger than 25 is _____ injuries, suicide, and _____.

25. Each plan of care must be _____ to a client's needs, age, and culture.

26. Urinary _____ is not a normal age-related change in the older adult.

EXERCISING YOUR CLINICAL JUDGMENT

27. Mr. Biaggio, the 42-year-old client from the chapter's case study, is struggling with balancing his roles as a husband, parent, and new employee. His children are in high school and plan to attend college in another state. He has become self-absorbed and distant from his family. Mr. Biaggio may be experiencing which psychosocial stage of development?
    1. Intimacy versus isolation
    2. Iindustry versus inferiority
    3. Integrity versus despair
    4. Generativity versus stagnation

28. Mr. Biaggio has been reviewing and re-evaluating his life including his life accomplishments. He has been experiencing inner turmoil and self-doubt. He is most likely experiencing:
    1. poor job performance.
    2. a situational crisis.
    3. a midlife crisis.
    4. poor family relationships.

29. To help persuade Mr. Biaggio to change his high-risk behaviors, you will need to:
    1. give Mr. Biaggio both oral and written health education material.
    2. have Mr. Biaggio join a support group made up of men his age.
    3. identify Mr. Biaggio's beliefs relevant to his high-risk behaviors and provide him information based on this foundation.
    4. give Mr. Biaggio your recommendations regarding his most serious high-risk behavior so he may begin working on modifying it.

TEST YOURSELF

30. Middle adulthood is the period from ages 35 to 64 when mature adults are concerned with:
    1. developing philosophies of life and personal lifestyles.
    2. balancing a career with raising small children.
    3. establishing a significant relationship with a partner.
    4. establishing and guiding the next generation in their roles as parents, teachers, mentors, guardians of the culture, etc.

31. Your client has a child in high school and is caring for his elderly parent. As a group, clients in this situation are often commonly called the:
    1. midlevel generation.
    2. x-generation.
    3. sandwich generation.
    4. midlife transition generation.

32. You are admitting a client to your health care facility. What is the most important thing you need to do to ensure that you obtain a thorough and accurate history of the client's problems?
    1. Read the client's admission record prior to your assessment.
    2. Develop a trusting relationship with the client.
    3. Obtain biographical data, history, and chief complaint.
    4. Obtain family history and chief complaint.

Copyright © 2004, Elsevier Science (USA). All Rights Reserved.

33. You should do which of the following diagnostic screening tests with your young adult clients?
    1. TB, vision, Papanicolaou smear, breast exam
    2. TB, prostate-specific antigen test, cholesterol
    3. BP, breast exam, prostate-specific antigen test
    4. TB, sigmoidoscopy, vision

34. Your assessment of your client, who is 20 years old, reveals that she has had several unwanted pregnancies, and abuses alcohol.
    Which nursing diagnosis would be most appropriate?
    1. *Ineffective health maintenance*
    2. *Knowledge deficit*
    3. *Ineffective management of therapeutic regimen*
    4. *Delayed growth and development*

35. Your client is involved in an adult day care program. This type of long-term-care service offers which of the following?
    1. Temporary respite for family caregivers by allowing a resident to live in assisted living community or nursing home
    2. Inpatient care designed for adults who have an acute illness, injury, or exacerbation of disease process
    3. Community-based group programs designed to meet the needs of functionally impaired adults through individualized plans of care
    4. Provides residents 24-hour nursing care available from licensed nurses

Copyright © 2004, Elsevier Science (USA). All Rights Reserved.

Health Perception

18

PURPOSE

This chapter discusses key concepts that relate to the nursing diagnosis *Health-seeking behaviors*. It provides you with definitions of health and describes the perception of health for individuals, families, and communities. In addition, this chapter identifies health goals and expected outcomes when planning care for individuals, families, and communities. It also discusses factors affecting health and interventions you can use to promote health.

MATCHING

1. ____disease
2. ____etiology
3. ____health goals
4. ____health-illness continuum
5. ____health perception
6. ____health promotion
7. ____health within illness
8. ____illness
9. ____longevity statistics
10. ____population health
11. ____preventive health care
12. ____primary health care
13. ____primary prevention
14. ____secondary prevention
15. ____tertiary prevention
16. ____well-being
17. ____wellness

a. knowledge and experience of one's state of wellness and well-being

b. refers to the personal experience of feeling unhealthy, caused by changes in a person's state of well-being and social function.

c. an event that can expand human potential by providing an opportunity for personal growth and well-being despite having an illness

d. the advancement of health through the encouragement of activities that enhance the wellness of individuals, families, and communities

e. a subjective perception of a good and satisfactory existence in which the individual has a positive experience of personal abilities, harmony, and vitality

f. considers health problems encountered as a result of being a part of a group and focuses intervention on the population rather than on the individual

g. a specific disorder characterized by a recognizable set of signs and symptoms and attributable to heredity, infection, diet, or environment

h. consists of actions that are considered true prevention because they precede disease or dysfunction and are applied to clients considered physically and emotionally healthy to protect them from health problems

i. outline broadly what needs to be done to achieve health for individuals, families, and communities

j. the cause of the disease

k. ranges from high-level wellness—an optimal state of mental and physical well-being—to premature death

l. consists of actions that focus on the early diagnosis and prompt treatment of people with health problems or illnesses and who are at risk for developing complications or worsening conditions

m. all care necessary to people's lives and health, including health education, nutrition, sanitation, maternal and child health care, immunizations, and prevention and control of endemic disease

n. life expectancy

Copyright © 2004, Elsevier Science (USA). All Rights Reserved.

o. recognition of the risk for disease and actions taken to reduce that risk

p. a state of optimal health or optimal physical and social functioning

q. involves minimizing the effects of a permanent irreversible disease or disability through interventions directed at preventing complication and deterioration

TRUE OR FALSE

18. ____Health perception is the knowledge and experience of one's state of wellness and well-being.

19. ____Countries around the world are seeking to establish and attain health goals for their citizens.

20. ____The World Health Organization (WHO) has declared that it is unrealistic to believe that health is a fundamental right of all people.

21. ____All diseases can be cured by removing their etiology.

22. ____Every person exists at some point on the health-illness continuum and may move back and forth between the two extremes.

23. ____ Population health is primarily concerned with public policies and interventions.

24. ____The key element of *Health-seeking behaviors* is choice.

25. ____Society at large is responsible for the health of its members.

FILL-IN-THE-BLANKS

26. The ____ ____ ____ has defined health as a state of complete physical, mental, and social well-being, and not merely the absence of illness.

27. The overarching goal of *Healthy People 2010* is increasing the ____ and ____ of healthy life.

28. Wellness is a ____ that cannot be ____ achieved.

29. Health care is the ____ and treatment of disease based on a specific disorder and its etiology.

30. The ____ ____ ____ recognizes that more than one factor is necessary to determine a person's state of health.

31. Health in a community is defined by the parameters of ____ health.

32. A statement of health goals flows from the ____ of health

33. Primary ____ care refers to care provided at the point at which a client first enters the health care system.

TEST YOURSELF

34. You are organizing a public forum to identify health goals for the local teen center. Your plan is to have teens actively seek ways to alter detrimental personal health habits so they can move toward a higher level of health. You are doing your health care planning based on the goals of *Healthy People 2010*. The overarching goals of *Healthy People 2010* include which of the following?
    1. To help individuals of all ages increase life expectancy and improve their quality of life and to eliminate health disparities among different segments of the population
    2. Essential health services must be available to all persons without regard to age, risk category, present health status, or ability to pay.
    3. Essential services should be planned, funded, and supervised on a nonprofit basis by public authorities.
    4. Essential health services should be available to those eligible when they are away from home.

35. When planning your assessment of the teen center, which broad social issues might you consider assessing?
    1. Whether it is a safe environment, and whether it offers cost-effective health services
    2. Whether individual teens have good relationships with their peers
    3. Whether the teens have good coping skills
    4. Whether individual teens have the capacity to make healthy lifestyle decisions

36. You are concerned about the high levels of depression in the teen population. You organize and screen the teens for depression. This type of prevention is:
    1. primary.
    2. secondary.
    3. tertiary.
    4. evaluation.

Copyright © 2004, Elsevier Science (USA). All Rights Reserved.

37. The World Health Organization (WHO) has defined health as:
    1. the absence of disease.
    2. a state of complete physical, mental, and social well-being.
    3. knowledge and experience of one's state of wellness and well-being.
    4. a state of complete physical, mental, and social well-being, and not merely the absence of disease.

38. When assessing community health, your nursing care plan may include which of the following broad social issues of community health?
    1. Positive, supportive interpersonal family relationships, safety and security issues, affordable housing
    2. Community design, joint action for minority and cultural health, social services, and public policy
    3. A safe environment, preventive health services, and consequences of lower-status occupations
    4. Access to and appropriate use of health care services, affordable housing, and a safe environment

39. Immunization programs are an example of which level of preventive care?
    1. Primary prevention
    2. Secondary prevention
    3. Tertiary prevention
    4. Disease prevention

Copyright © 2004, Elsevier Science (USA). All Rights Reserved.

Health Maintenance: Lifestyle Management

PURPOSE

This chapter introduces you to worldviews of health, health care, and behavior change that affect one's decisions about lifestyle changes as part of a therapeutic regimen. It helps you to use the nursing process when working with clients seeking to make these lifestyle changes to enhance health and well-being.

MATCHING

1. ____ action stage
2. ____ contemplation stage
3. ____ counseling
4. ____ emic dimension
5. ____ etic dimension
6. ____ lifestyle
7. ____ maintenance stage
8. ____ perceived barriers
9. ____ perceived benefits
10. ____ perceived severity
11. ____ perceived susceptibility
12. ____ precontemplation stage
13. ____ preparation stage
14. ____ referral
15. ____ self-efficacy
16. ____ social support
17. ____ termination stage

a. person's subjective perception of the risk of contracting a health condition.

b. the person does not intend to change a high-risk behavior in the foreseeable future (the next 6 months), primarily because he or she is unaware of the long-term consequences of the behavior

c. perceived negative aspects of a health action or the perceived impediments to undertaking the recommended behaviors

d. the person changes risky behaviors and the context of the behavior (environment, experience) and makes significant efforts to reach goals

e. the perceived seriousness of contracting an illness or leaving it untreated

f. the person intends to change within the next 6 months

g. the conviction that one can successfully execute the behavior required to produce the outcomes

h. takes place during the 6 months after the person changes the high-risk behavior

i. refers to an individual's or social group's subjective perceptions and experiences related to health

j. the subjective feeling of belonging, or being accepted, loved, esteemed, valued, and needed for oneself, not for what one can do for others

k. a behavior or group of behaviors chosen by the person that may have a positive or a negative influence on health

l. a process designed to provide the client with access to health care and supportive services that are not available form the sending institution

m. refers to the objective interpretation of health by a scientifically trained practitioner

n. the person is no longer tempted to engage in old behavior

Copyright © 2004, Elsevier Science (USA). All Rights Reserved.

o. a method of communication that actively involves the client in the recognition of personal risk factors and management of necessary behavior changes

p. the person's perceptions and beliefs about the effectiveness of the recommended actions in preventing the health threat

q. the person intends to take action in the very near future, usually within the next month

TRUE OR FALSE

18. ____ To effectively help others, health care professionals must first understand the impact of their own beliefs about health on the health practices of their clients.

19. ____ According to the health belief model, clients will take action to control ill health if the anticipated barriers to taking the action are outweighed by the benefits.

20. ____ Impaired verbal skills or language differences do not interfere with the ability of a client to effectively express health needs to health care professionals.

21. ____ Clients with health insurance are more likely to seek health care at the onset of symptoms than those who do not have insurance.

22. ____ A client's spiritual values and beliefs always coincide with recommended interventions to promote, maintain, or restore health.

23. ____ The nursing diagnosis *Noncompliance* is used when a client desires to comply but factors are present that deter adherence to health-related advice given by health professionals.

24. ____ Counseling is different from education in that counseling involves guiding the client through decision making rather than merely providing the information needed to make a decision.

25. ____ A nurse should anticipate problems in managing the therapeutic regimen if the client has poor eyesight, decreased mobility, or reduced manual dexterity.

26. ____ The nurse is solely responsible for the discharge planning process.

27. ____ If no noticeable change occurs in unhealthy behaviors within a reasonable time, the client should be reassessed to determine what prevented progress.

FILL-IN-THE-BLANKS

28. The theory of_____ _____ is a human behavior framework designed to explain a person's intention to perform a behavior.

29. Health practices and behaviors that have potential negative effects on health are known as _____ _____.

30. A health-risk appraisal provides clients with essential information about health threats from hereditary factors, _____, and _____ history.

31. The client with a nursing diagnosis of *Health-seeking behaviors* does not necessarily have a _____ diagnosis.

32. A nurse who provides specific information to a client about a health problem in order to motivate health behavior is striving to increase the client's _____ level.

33. _____ _____ is a self-discovery process that may be helpful in assisting a client to make health-related choices when faced with one or more alternatives.

34. Building rewards into effective management of the health care regimen is a method of providing _____ or _____ factors.

35. A client who is in _____ is not likely to see the need for or benefit of health care services that are provided through referral.

36. _____ planning begins at the time of admission, but should be finalized with a specific plan before the client leaves an institution.

37. The assistance of family and friends in facilitating health-related behavioral change is considered a type of _____ support.

EXERCISING YOUR CLINICAL JUDGMENT

Mr. Kitchener, the African-American man identified in the chapter case study, has a nursing diagnosis of *Ineffective therapeutic regimen management*. His identified health problem is heart failure and he was prescribed digoxin (a cardiac glycoside), Hygroton (a thiazide diuretic), and Lasix (a loop diuretic) at his first clinic visit. Mr. Kitchener did not return to the clinic when he was scheduled for a follow-up appointment, but came today after experiencing a return of shortness of breath. He had stopped taking his medication because he felt better, and because he disliked having to go to the bathroom so frequently. Recall that he is a widower with no family nearby, and he does not carefully plan meals or

Copyright © 2004, Elsevier Science (USA). All Rights Reserved.

attend to his health. He also is a smoker who is not motivated as yet to stop smoking. You have been asked by the clinic nurse to provide teaching to Mr. Kitchener to enhance his ability to manage his health problems at home.

38. If Mr. Kitchener does not yet perceive that there are health benefits from smoking cessation, you would determine that he is in which of the following stages in the transtheoretical model of behavior change?
    1. Precontemplation
    2. Contemplation
    3. Preparation
    4. Action

39. Which of the following factors is most likely to be responsible for Mr. Kitchener's lack of adherence to the medical regimen?
    1. Complexity of the therapeutic regimen
    2. Side effects of therapy
    3. Financial cost of the regimen
    4. Complexity of the health care delivery system

40. The most effective strategy to use when providing information to Mr. Kitchener about his health problem would be to:
    1. explain that he will have a steady downhill course if he does not adhere to the treatment plan.
    2. share with him the results of research studies that show the cost of treating other noncompliant clients who have similar health problems.
    3. increase his awareness that unhealthy lifestyle habits are related to the development of his symptoms.
    4. encourage him to hire a companion to cook his meals and make sure he takes his medication.

41. You realize that Mr. Kitchener needs supportive care in order to achieve and maintain lifestyle changes. Given this client's particular situation, you would select which of the following as the most important intervention for this client?
    1. Make referrals to all available services that are provided within the clinic setting.
    2. Contact other outside agencies to give follow-up care.
    3. Ask him to renew his relationships with family that lives out of town.
    4. Establish a trusting therapeutic relationship with him.

TEST YOURSELF

42. To improve overall health, the nurse would place highest priority on assisting the client to make lifestyle changes for which of the following habits?
    1. Drinking a six-pack of beer each day
    2. Eating an occasional chocolate bar
    3. Exercising twice a week
    4. Using relaxation exercises to deal with stress

43. A nurse who is assessing the health-related physical fitness of a client as part of a health assessment would focus on which of the following aspects of the assessment?
    1. Agility
    2. Speed
    3. Body composition
    4. Power

44. A nurse would interpret that which of the following clients is most likely to have a reduced ability to acquire knowledge about a newly prescribed diet and medication regimen due to cognitive perceptual impairment?
    1. One who has a slight decrease in hearing acuity
    2. One who has chronic confusion
    3. One who wears corrective lenses
    4. One who is 48 years old

45. A client with a newly diagnosed health problem has the choice of using either of two acceptable treatments for the problem. If the client has difficulty choosing between the two, the nurse would consider which of the following nursing diagnoses as most appropriate?
    1. *Health-seeking behaviors*
    2. *Knowledge deficit*
    3. *Ineffective health maintenance*
    4. *Decisional conflict*

46. A nurse is trying to motivate a client toward more effective management of a therapeutic regimen. Which of the following actions by the nurse is most likely to be effective in increasing the client's motivation?
    1. Determine whether the client has any family or friends living nearby.
    2. Develop a lengthy discharge plan and review it carefully with the client.
    3. Teach the client about the disorder at the client's level of understanding.
    4. Make a referral to an area agency for client follow-up.

Copyright © 2004, Elsevier Science (USA). All Rights Reserved.

Health Maintenance: Medication Management

PURPOSE

This chapter describes concepts of medication management and a wide variety of factors that can influence the effectiveness of medication therapy. It provides specific guidelines and information related to nursing process that can assist you to effectively deliver medication therapy to clients.

MATCHING

1. ____ adverse effect

2. ____ anaphylaxis

3. ____ antagonistic effect

4. ____ bioavailability

5. ____ biotransformation

6. ____ controlled substance

7. ____ generic name

8. ____ hypersensitivity reaction

9. ____ idiosyncratic response

10. ____ intradermal route

11. ____ intramuscular route

12. ____ intravenous route

13. ____ loading dose

14. ____ official name

15. ____ parenteral route

16. ____ pharmacokinetics

17. ____ prescription

18. ____ side effect

19. ____ subcutaneous route

20. ____ synergistic effect

21. ____ target organ

22. ____ teratogenic potential

23. ____ therapeutic effect

24. ____ topical route

25. ____ toxic effect

26. ____ trade name

a. the amount of an administered drug that is available for activity in the target tissue

b. a mild allergic reaction to a drug

c. involves injection into the subcutaneous tissue just under the dermis

d. a medication side effect that is potentially harmful to a client

e. involves injection of a medication into a vein

f. the likelihood that a medication will harm a developing fetus

g. refers to a drug's activity from the time it enters the body until it leaves

h. a serious adverse effect of a medication that may even threaten life

i. an effect that occurs when one drug enhances or increases the effect of another drug

j. a body tissue or organ that is specifically affected by a drug

k. an unexplained and unpredictable response to a medication

l. the name assigned to a drug when it is first manufactured; also known as the nonproprietary name

m. involves injection into muscle tissue, specifically the body of a muscle

Copyright © 2004, Elsevier Science (USA). All Rights Reserved.

n. an effect of a medication that is not intended or planned but may occur as a result of use

o. drug that affects the mind or behavior, may be habit forming, and has a high potential for abuse

p. an effect that occurs when one drug reduces or negates the effect of another

q. an initial medication dose that exceeds the maintenance or therapeutic dose

r. the intended effect or action of a medication

s. used to deliver medication directly into a body site, such as skin, eyes, or ears

t. the name assigned by the Food and Drug Administration (FDA) after it approves a drug; often the same name as the generic name

u. involves injection into the dermis

v. an order for a medication that contains the client's name, medication name, dose, route, frequency, amount of medication to be dispensed, and the number of refills allowed

w. a copyrighted name given by a specific manufacturer to a medication; also known as the brand name or proprietary name

x. a drug route that is outside the GI tract

y. the process of inactivating and breaking down a medication

z. a life-threatening allergic reaction to a drug that requires immediate intervention to prevent possible death

TRUE OR FALSE

27. ____In some states, revised Nurse Practice Acts have allowed selected groups of advanced practice nurses to write prescriptions.

28. ____The blood-brain barrier permits transport of lipid-bound medications while preventing transport of many water-soluble drugs.

29. ____No drug reaches the liver until it has passed through all body tissues.

30. ____The peak serum concentration of a medication usually occurs just as the last bit of the most recently administered dose is being absorbed.

31. ____There is a national standard recognized throughout all states that regulates how and when telephone and verbal medication orders should be given.

32. ____The most common medication system in use today is the unit-dose system.

33. ____A client's overall nutritional status can either positively or negatively affect medication actions in the body.

34. ____Dehydration has no effect on drug transport because the dosage is unchanged.

35. ____A client who subscribes to Western beliefs about health and illness typically expects to receive medication as part of the treatment plan.

FILL-IN-THE-BLANKS

36. In the United States the _____ _____ Agency is empowered to enforce narcotic laws.

37. _____ _____ refers to the diminishing therapeutic effect of the same dosage of a drug over time, requiring increased dosing to achieve the same therapeutic effect.

38. _____-_____ drugs are coated to prevent them from dissolving until they reach the alkaline environment of the small intestine.

39. A drug that should be avoided during pregnancy because the risks outweigh any benefits is labeled as belonging to FDA Pregnancy Risk Category _____.

40. Drug dosages for infants and children are calculated according to either body surface area or _____ _____.

41. Nursing diagnoses that could apply due to the gastrointestinal side effects of medications include _____ and _____.

42. A client who develops signs such as oral lesions, diarrhea, or vaginal itching while taking antibiotic therapy could be developing _____.

43. In many agencies, a medication should be administered within _____ minutes before or after its scheduled time.

EXERCISING YOUR CLINICAL JUDGMENT

Mr. Connell, the 62-year-old Irish-American introduced in the chapter case study, has high blood pressure, but stopped taking prescribed medications because he "felt better." He has been treated in the local hospital emergency department for chest pain and is now diagnosed with angina pectoris. You must teach Mr. Connell about the medications that are being resumed.

Copyright © 2004 Elsevier Science (USA). All Rights Reserved.

44. Which of the following items would you include in a discussion with Mr. Connell about general principles of medication self-administration?
    1. If the prescription runs out, use that of a relative or friend until it can be refilled.
    2. Change brand names depending on cost to motivate compliance with therapy.
    3. Develop and use a reminder system if forgetting medications is a problem.
    4. Put all types of medications into a single large container to make storage easier.

45. You are teaching Mr. Connell strategies to prevent dizziness, a common side effect of antihypertensive medications. Which of the following would you recommend?
    1. Use alcohol at will because it adds to the antihypertensive effect.
    2. Sit or stand up slowly when getting out of a bed or chair.
    3. Go out for long walks in hot weather for additive medication effects.
    4. Take the medication upon arising in the morning if dizziness is a chronic problem.

46. Which of the following directions would you give Mr. Connell about taking nitroglycerin because it is a sublingual medication?
    1. Chew the tablet thoroughly
    2. Swallow it whole
    3. Place it between the cheek and the gum
    4. Let it dissolve under the tongue

47. You would be careful to teach Mr. Connell about adverse medication effects knowing that he has an increased likelihood of experiencing these because of which of the following personal factors?
    1. Age
    2. Work history
    3. Medical diagnosis
    4. Cultural background

TEST YOURSELF

48. A client is exhibiting a toxic effect from a medication. Which of the following actions by the nurse is most appropriate?
    1. Withhold the dose and report the signs and symptoms to the prescriber.
    2. Administer half the dose for the next 3 days.
    3. Withhold the dose for 24 hours, then resume.
    4. Administer the next dose, but keep an antidote nearby

49. A client has an order for an intramuscular injection. The nurse selects an appropriate size syringe with which of the following needle lengths?
    1. $\frac{1}{2}$ to $\frac{5}{8}$ inch
    2. $\frac{5}{8}$ to 1 inch
    3. 1 to $1\frac{1}{2}$ inches
    4. $1\frac{1}{2}$ to 2 inches

50. A client has a new order for a transdermal patch. Which of the following would the nurse teach the client about maintaining safety with this type of medication?
    1. Apply the patch on a hairy site to prolong absorption.
    2. Use firm pressure, especially around the edges to ensure good skin contact.
    3. If a patch falls off, leave it off until the next day.
    4. Trim the patch so it fits under clothing without being visible.

51. A client is due for a dose of a scheduled eyedrop. Which of the following would the nurse do to safely administer this medication?
    1. Have the client lower the chin.
    2. Ask the client to look down at the floor.
    3. Tell the client to squint or squeeze the eye shut after administration.
    4. Pull downward on the bony orbit to expose the lower conjunctival sac.

52. A client has an order to take 5 ml of a medication at each dose. The home health nurse tells the client that this amount is equal to which of the following household measurements?
    1. $\frac{1}{2}$ teaspoon
    2. 1 teaspoon
    3. 2 teaspoons
    4. 1 tablespoon

Copyright © 2004, Elsevier Science (USA). All Rights Reserved.

Health Protection: Risk for Infection

PURPOSE

This chapter introduces you to the health problem of infection and the importance of infection control as it relates to nursing practice. It uses the nursing process as a framework in describing how to assess, diagnose, plan, implement, and evaluate strategies used to either prevent or treat infection.

MATCHING

1. ____ antibiotic
2. ____ antibody
3. ____ antimicrobial
4. ____ bacterium
5. ____ differential cell count
6. ____ Gram stain
7. ____ immunization
8. ____ immunosuppression
9. ____ infection
10. ____ inflammatory response
11. ____ isolation
12. ____ medical asepsis
13. ____ nosocomial infection
14. ____ pathogen
15. ____ septicemia
16. ____ standard precautions
17. ____ surgical asepsis
18. ____ virulence
19. ____ virus

a. a small single-celled organism that can reproduce outside cells

b. a clinical syndrome caused by the invasion and multiplication of a pathogen

c. a set of actions, including performing hand hygiene and the use of barriers, designed to reduce transmission of infectious organisms

d. consists of practices designed to reduce the numbers of pathogenic microorganisms in the client's environment

e. having the ability to limit the spread of microorganisms

f. a tiny microorganism, much smaller than a bacterium, that can only replicate inside the cell of a host such as a human

g. infection in the bloodstream

h. a circulating protein that recognizes and destroys foreign invaders or immunoglobulins

i. a drug that kills bacteria

j. an infection acquired from a reservoir in the hospital that may also be resistant to several antibiotics

k. breaks down the number of white blood cells into their types

l. a disease-producing microorganism

m. a localized reaction to injury that is activated when there is tissue damage

n. a specific microscopic test used to obtain rapid results on a culture sent to the laboratory

o. identification of a client who has an infection and implementation of precautions to prevent the spread of that infection

Copyright © 2004, Elsevier Science (USA). All Rights Reserved.

p. a medication administered to activate an immune response before exposure to the disease agent

q. suppression of the body's immune system

r. the power of an organism to cause disease

s. the protection of the client against infection before, during, and after surgery using sterile technique

TRUE OR FALSE

20. ____ The incubation period of an infection extends from the time of a client's first exposure to the organism to the appearance of the first symptoms.

21. ____ Virulence is a measure of the aggressiveness of an organism in causing a disease.

22. ____ Measles is an example of an infection that is carried by a vector.

23. ____ An individual's level of immunity is age-related.

24. ____ People with dementia are at increased risk of infection due to impaired protective responses.

25. ____ The presence of an increased number of immature neutrophils, which can indicate infection, is sometimes called a right shift.

26. ____ A Gram stain tests the nature of bacterial cell walls by determining whether they take up a stain.

27. ____ A person's state of anxiety has no effect on one's protection against infection.

28. ____ Contact precautions involve use of standard precautions plus the use of barrier items such as gloves and gowns.

29. ____ Minor cuts and bruises should be washed with mild soap and water and patted dry.

FILL-IN-THE-BLANKS

30. The period of _____ is the time following the height of the acute symptoms to the time the person experiences a return to normal health.

31. A place where an infectious agent can survive and possibly multiply until it can invade a susceptible host is called a _____.

32. _____ infections are those that result from organisms that do not ordinarily cause disease.

33. An _____ factor that contributes to increased risk of infection is overcrowded living conditions.

34. Redness, swelling, pain, and heat are signs that accompany a _____ infection.

35. The sink and bathroom of a hospital room are generally considered to be _____ areas.

36. Gloves should never be used as a substitute for good _____.

37. The _____ sterilization method kills microorganisms that are sensitive to heat and moisture.

38. Enteric precautions are designed to prevent disease transmission through direct or indirect contact with _____.

39. _____ precautions refer to precautions used for organisms that can be spread through the air but are unable to remain in the air for distances greater than 3 feet.

EXERCISING YOUR CLINICAL JUDGMENT

Luisa Martinez, the 6-month-old Mexican-American infant introduced in this chapter, is admitted with dehydration and possible sepsis following upper respiratory infection. Luisa lives with her parents, two older siblings, and her uncle and his entire family. Her father speaks and understands English, but her mother does not. You are assigned to care for Luisa while she is hospitalized.

40. You would expect to note which of the following signs of systemic infection while caring for Luisa?
    1. Malaise
    2. Redness
    3. Swelling
    4. Pain

41. When considering what to teach Luisa's parents about reducing the risk of further infection, you would begin with which of the following health practices?
    1. Food storage
    2. Food preparation
    3. Performing hand hygiene
    4. Bathing

42. If Luisa had been found to have a viral infection, such as influenza, as the basis for her symptoms, which of the following types of isolation would be important to implement in her care?
    1. Airborne
    2. Droplet
    3. Contact
    4. Strict

Copyright © 2004, Elsevier Science (USA). All Rights Reserved.

43. Luisa is started on antibiotic therapy to treat her infection. If she still had general malaise and fever after 7 days of therapy, the nurse would evaluate that which of the following would be the most likely follow-up?
    1. Increase her fluid intake.
    2. Change the antibiotic to an antiviral agent.
    3. Send her home because hospitalization didn't help.
    4. Reculture her throat and blood.

TEST YOURSELF

44. A nurse who is reviewing the medical record of a client would expect that the client has some type of infection if the results of the white blood cell count differential showed which of the following?
    1. Increased immature neutrophils
    2. Decreased monocytes
    3. Increased eosinophils
    4. Decreased basophils

45. The nurse is performing hand hygiene as part of medical asepsis. Which of the following nursing actions for rinsing the hands represents correct practice?
    1. Hands lower than elbows, water washing down hands to fingertips
    2. Hands lower than elbows, water washing from fingertips to wrists
    3. Hands higher than elbows, water washing down hands to fingertips
    4. Hands higher than elbows, water washing from fingertips to wrists

46. A client admitted with tuberculosis should be placed in isolation in which of the following rooms on the nursing unit?
    1. A two-bed room
    2. A four-bed room
    3. A private room with windows that open
    4. A private room with negative pressure

47. A home health nurse would provide client teaching about how to prevent infection in the home after noting which of the following?
    1. Sink and bathroom are clean
    2. Leftover cooked food is stored on countertop
    3. Individuals perform hand hygiene before touching food
    4. Individuals use tissues when sneezing

48. A nurse has an order to change a dressing using sterile technique. After opening a package of sterile gloves, the nurse would do which of the following first to put them on correctly?
    1. Grasp the glove from the inside edge
    2. Grasp the glove from the outside edge
    3. Grasp the folded edge of the cuff
    4. Grasp it anywhere desired

Copyright © 2004, Elsevier Science (USA). All Rights Reserved.

Health Protection: Risk for Injury

PURPOSE

This chapter introduces you to concepts of injury and internal and external factors that are associated with increased risk. It uses nursing process as a framework to help you identify nursing actions that can help prevent injury and those that can minimize risk of further injury.

MATCHING

1. ____aspiration

2. ____burns

3. ____choking

4. ____injury

5. ____poisoning

6. ____restraint

7. ____strangulation

8. ____suffocation

9. ____trauma

a. an internal obstruction of the airway by food or a foreign body

b. an interruption in breathing that results from a severe lack of oxygen (asphyxia) where there is no source of air, an inadequate supply of oxygen in the air, or a condition in which the air cannot be inhaled

c. a physical injury or wound caused by a forceful, disruptive, or violent action

d. constriction of the airway from an external cause

e. any injuries caused by excessive exposure to electricity, chemicals, gases, radioactivity, or thermal agents

f. the inspiration of foreign material into the airway

g. a device intended for medical purposes that limits movement to the extent necessary for treatment, examination, or protection of the client

h. trauma or damage to some part of the body

i. an adverse condition or physical state resulting from the administration of a toxic substance

TRUE OR FALSE

10. ____Injury can result from physical, mechanical, biological, or chemical agents.

11. ____The biggest concern when an older adult falls is the threat of a hip fracture.

12. ____Faulty electrical equipment is the leading cause of fatal residential fires.

13. ____Older adults are at increased risk of fire death because they are more vulnerable to smoke inhalation and burns and are less likely to recover.

14. ____A single, stressful lifting event is the cause of most back injuries.

15. ____A person's lifestyle can raise the risk of injury.

16. ____Potential hazards in the home are inadequate lighting, missing or broken steps or handrails, or the presence of throw rugs.

17. ____A person's cognitive and perceptual abilities are crucial to promoting safety.

18. ____All child car seats should be bought based on the child's weight and height.

19. ____Substance abuse can reduce a person's judgment and coordination and the ability to complete typical tasks.

Copyright © 2004, Elsevier Science (USA). All Rights Reserved.

FILL-IN-THE-BLANKS

20. Accidents that most commonly result in death include motor vehicle accidents and _____.

21. Clients who are unconscious from drugs or alcohol, or who have a cerebrovascular accident or cardiac arrest are at risk for _____.

22. _____ can enter the body through ingestion, inhalation, injection, application, or absorption of the noxious material.

23. Motor vehicle accidents are the leading cause of _____ deaths in the United States.

24. Potential _____ hazards to safety may result from noise, dust, air pollution, working with dangerous machinery, or being exposed to toxic substances.

25. A frequently cited reason for ignoring safety is a lack of _____.

26. Clients at the developmental levels of _____ and _____ are particularly vulnerable to accidents and injuries because of their limited awareness of potential dangers.

27. When planning care for a client with an increased risk for injury, the nurse should focus primarily on _____.

28. The nurse can help prevent electrical shocks by using equipment that is electrically _____.

29. The acronym RACE used in fire safety stands for _____, _____, _____, and _____.

EXERCISING YOUR CLINICAL JUDGMENT

Juanita Soto, a 75-year-old widow with rheumatoid arthritis who lives alone, is being followed by a home health nurse due to declining mobility and partial loss of vision. She recently fell and required a brief hospitalization.

30. Which of the following factors in Mrs. Soto's physical environment places her at risk for further falls?
    1. Intact stairs with treads
    2. Throw rugs on tile floors
    3. Night light in hallway
    4. Grab bars in bathroom

31. The home health nurse would reinforce to Mrs. Soto that she should do which of the following to prevent becoming burned in the home setting?
    1. Leave electrical outlets uncovered for ease of use.
    2. Keep pot handles facing the back of the stove.
    3. Use an open-flame heater for added warmth in cold weather.
    4. Use extension cords to be able to maximize ability to use electric plugs.

32. The nurse assesses Mrs. Soto for physiological risk factors for falls. The nurse would conclude that she is at no further risk if which of the following were discovered?
    1. History of dizziness
    2. Need for wheelchair due to reduced mobility
    3. Weakness and fatigue noted when climbing stairs
    4. Intact recent and remote memory

33. The nurse notes that Mrs. Soto has no fire extinguisher in the home. Which of the following types of fire extinguishers should be recommended?
    1. Water pump extinguisher (type A)
    2. Foam extinguisher (type B)
    3. Multipurpose extinguisher (types A, B, C)
    4. Dry powder extinguisher (type D)

TEST YOURSELF

34. When a nurse is working with older adults in the hospital, the nurse should assess each client for risk for falls. If the nurse assesses the client as having medium risk for falling while hospitalized, which one of the following would be true about the client?
    1. Has periods of confusion; noncompliance with safety measures
    2. Ambulates with a steady gait, can perform self-care activities without assistance, cognitively intact
    3. Needs some assistance when performing certain daily activities, alert, cooperative; may have a chronic physical alignment that could her from calling for help
    4. Denies obvious problems of ambulation or mobility; may refuse to call for assistance

35. The nurse working with a population of clients of all ages would interpret that which of the following clients has the least risk of poisoning?
    1. Toddlers
    2. Young children
    3. Older adults with sensory impairment
    4. Young adults

36. After calling the poison control center, an ambulatory care nurse prepares to induce vomiting in a client being seen with overdose. The nurse should select which of the following as the agent of choice?
    1. Activated charcoal
    2. Syrup of ipecac
    3. Hypertonic saline
    4. Any solution containing phosphate

Copyright © 2004, Elsevier Science (USA). All Rights Reserved.

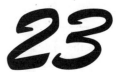

Promoting Healthy Nutrition

PURPOSE

This chapter discusses key concepts that relate to normal nutrition. It provides an overview of how you will use the nursing process to assist clients in maintaining and/or improving nutritional health.

MATCHING

1. ____ amino acids

2. ____ anthropometric measurements

3. ____ calorie

4. ____ carbohydrates

5. ____ disaccharides

6. ____ fiber

7. ____ glycogen

8. ____ metabolism

9. ____ minerals

10. ____ monosaccharides

11. ____ nutrient

12. ____ nutrition

13. ____ nutritional status

14. ____ polysaccharide

15. ____ proteins

16. ____ recommended dietary allowance (RDA)

17. ____ starch

18. ____ triglycerides

19. ____ vitamins

a. measurements of physical characteristics of the body (such as height and weight), as well as the amount of muscle tissue or fat tissue in the body

b. simple or complex compounds composed of carbon, oxygen, and hydrogen

c. the form in which carbohydrates are stored in humans and in meat

d. a measure of the energy content of food

e. a biochemical substance utilized by the body for growth, maintenance, and repair

f. the condition of the body resulting from the use of essential nutrients available to it

g. subunits of carbohydrates that are six-carbon sugars (glucose, fructose, and galactose are examples)

h. compounds containing polymers of amino acids, linked together in a chain to form polypeptide bonds

i. compounds composed of carbon, hydrogen, oxygen, and an amino group that are classified as essential or nonessential, depending on whether the body can manufacture them from other sources

j. the level of a nutrient that is adequate to meet the needs of almost all healthy people, as determined by the Food and Nutrition Board of the National Research Council

k. organic substances found in food that serve as coenzymes in enzymatic reactions

l. composed of three fatty acids and a glycol unit; the chief form of fat in the diet and the main form of fat transport in the blood

m. the process by which energy from nutrients can be used by the cells or stored for later use

n. inorganic elements that are present in small amounts in virtually all body fluids and tissues

o. a group of monosaccharides joined together in a chain; they can be converted back to monosaccharides through a process called acid hydrolysis

p. the form in which plants store glucose

q. the structure of which plants are composed; includes cellulose, hemicellulose, pectins, gums, and mucilages

Copyright © 2004, Elsevier Science (USA). All Rights Reserved.

r. the science of food and nutrients, and the processes by which an organism takes them in and uses them for energy to grow, maintain function, and renew itself

s. molecules that form when two monosaccharides condense and join together to form a double sugar

TRUE OR FALSE

20. ____ A woman who is pregnant has an increased need for iron, calcium, and other vitamins.

21. ____ Most enzymatic digestion and virtually all absorption occur in the large intestine.

22. ____ The chemical energy from food is converted by the body to electrical, thermal, or mechanical energy, depending on the needs of the body.

23. ____ A diet high in fiber contains foods such as cereals, meats, and poultry.

24. ____ When the body is storing protein, negative nitrogen balance and catabolism occur.

25. ____ When taking medications, it is important to note whether there are foods that can cause drug-nutrient reactions.

26. ____ During pregnancy the need for both calorie and fluid intake increases.

27. ____ Taking in the RDA of a nutrient will meet the body's needs for that nutrient regardless of whether the client is well or ill.

28. ____ Body composition can be determined by measuring the triceps fat fold and midarm muscle circumference.

29. ____ Eating a diet high in calories and fat or eating late at night are likely characteristics of a client with the nursing diagnosis *Imbalanced nutrition: more than body requirements.*

30. ____ Antioxidants are found in yellow and red and green leafy vegetables.

FILL-IN-THE-BLANKS

31. _____ is the process by which the body changes food into elemental nutrients that can be absorbed.

32. Cellulose, pectins, gums, and mucilages are examples of _____.

33. As energy sources, both protein and carbohydrates provide _____ calories per gram.

34. _____ are organic substances found in food that serve as coenzymes in enzymatic reactions.

35. Zinc, iron, copper, and selenium are examples of _____.

36. Analysis of the type and amount of food eaten by a client is done by taking a _____.

37. Teaching clients about the type and number of food servings to eat each day can be done using the _____ _____ _____.

38. Albumin and prealbumin levels are indicators of _____ intake.

39. As a health promotion measure, nurses should teach clients to read the _____ _____ _____ _____ that must appear on all manufactured food products.

40. The second level of the Food Guide Pyramid includes _____ and _____.

41. _____ are plant compounds found in foods such as red wine, tea, apples, grapes, and may reduce the risk of heart disease and cancer.

EXERCISING YOUR CLINICAL JUDGEMENT

Mr. Crane is a 76-year-old man living alone in his own home. He has a son and daughter-in-law who live in the area. During a routine health visit, he tells the nurse in the physician's office that he has not been very interested in food following the death of his wife (who did most of the cooking) 2 months ago. The nurse notes that Mr. Crane has lost 7 pounds since his last visit 3 months ago, and has a current weight of 149 pounds (at the low end of the normal range for a man of his size). He can drive to the grocery store, but has limited income to spend on food. He has dentures that seem to fit well, but has a history of arthritis in the hands and knees.

42. The nurse would determine that which of the following factors is a positive one, which does not negatively influence Mr. Crane's nutritional status?
    1. Difficulty in using the hands
    2. Financial concerns
    3. Ability to chew and swallow
    4. Decreased appetite secondary to grief

43. The nurse interprets that Mr. Crane's arthritis of the hands would be which of the following types of barriers to adequate nutrition?
    1. Psychological
    2. Physical
    3. Cultural
    4. Financial

Copyright © 2004, Elsevier Science (USA). All Rights Reserved.

44. If Mr. Crane indicates an interest in obtaining help with shopping and/or food preparation, the nurse should first investigate which of the following resources?
    1. Ability of the son and daughter-in-law to help
    2. Private housekeeper
    3. Meals-on-Wheels delivery service
    4. Ability to use a microwave oven

45. In providing teaching to Mr. Crane about the elements of a healthy diet, the nurse would find which of the following to be the most helpful resource to use during the information session?
    1. Recommended Dietary Allowances chart
    2. Nutrition book
    3. Textbook on aging
    4. Food Guide Pyramid chart

TEST YOURSELF

46. A nurse who is teaching clients about lowering risk of hypertension (high blood pressure) would emphasize limiting which of the following types of substances in the daily diet?
    1. Salt
    2. Sugar
    2. Fiber
    3. Seeds and nuts

47. Although fats should be used sparingly in the diet, the nurse would encourage the use of which of the following types of fats when fat is needed during food preparation?
    1. Monounsaturated
    2. Polyunsaturated
    3. Hydrogenated
    4. Saturated

48. A prepubescent child has an increased need for calcium in the diet. The school nurse would teach children of this age group to increase intake of which of the following types of foods to obtain this nutrient?
    1. Meats
    3. Fish
    3. Raw fruits
    4. Dairy products

49. The nurse would encourage a client who is pregnant to take which of the following dietary supplements that cannot be met sufficiently with proper daily diet?
    1. Vitamin C and the B vitamins
    2. Vitamins A and D
    3. Ferrous iron and folacin
    4. Iron and magnesium

50. The nurse teaching clients about intake of high-fiber foods to protect against colorectal cancer would encourage the use of which of the following types of foods in the meal plan?
    1. Cooked fruits
    2. Cruciferous vegetables
    3. Lean meats
    4. Products made with refined flour

51. A female client asks about foods to eat that will provide a good source of phytoestrogen. Which of the following foods would the nurse recommend?
    1. Soy products
    2. Red meat
    3. Yellow vegetables
    4. Citrus fruits

Copyright © 2004, Elsevier Science (USA). All Rights Reserved.

Restoring Nutrition

PURPOSE

This chapter introduces you to nutritional deficits such as malnutrition and starvation, and the factors that aid in their development. It guides you in the use of the nursing process to facilitate optimum nutrition for clients with a nutritional deficit.

MATCHING

1. ____ anorexia

2. ____ catabolism

3. ____ deglutition

4. ____ dysphagia

5. ____ enteral nutrition

6. ____ malnutrition

7. ____ parenteral nutrition

a. the reflex passage of food, fluids, or both from the mouth to the stomach

b. any disorder of nutrition caused by unbalanced, insufficient, or excessive diet or from impaired absorption or metabolism of nutrients

c. the provision of total nutrition through a central or peripheral intravenous catheter

d. loss of appetite

e. the breakdown of muscle and lean body mass when nutrient intake fails to meet energy expenditure

f. difficulty in swallowing

g. any form of nutrition delivered to the gastrointestinal tract, although commonly used to refer to tube feedings

TRUE OR FALSE

8. ____ Nutritional deprivation can occur with problems that raise energy needs, such as infection, trauma, stress, or surgery.

9. ____ If a client has been starving for a period of time, the urine will be negative for ketones and nitrogen balance will be positive.

10. ____ Kwashiorkor is a condition of starvation caused by decreased protein intake, and usually occurs in young children after weaning.

11. ____ Marasmus is a condition of starvation that results from deficient caloric intake over a very short period of time.

12. ____ Bleeding tendencies can be associated with a deficiency of vitamin K.

13. ____ Approximately half of clients aged 65 and older wear dentures, which can affect nutritional intake.

14. ____ Changes in appetite include anorexia, early satiety, lack of interest in food, and loss of taste.

15. ____ A weight gain program is generally considered successful if the client gains at least 5 pounds per month.

16. ____ Food intake can be enhanced by serving meals in an attractive manner and making the environment as pleasant as possible.

17. ____ A client who is diabetic should be allowed small amounts of concentrated sweets.

FILL-IN-THE-BLANKS

18. Involuntary control of swallowing is coordinated in the lower pons and the _____ of the brain.

19. Pernicious anemia results from a deficiency of vitamin _____.

20. Anemia is most commonly associated with reduced intake of _____.

21. Premature infants may require tube feedings because the suck-swallow reflex does not develop until _____ weeks of gestation.

Copyright © 2004, Elsevier Science (USA). All Rights Reserved.

22. Serum studies are often ordered to evaluate a client who has unintentionally lost _____ % of his or her weight during the past 6 months.

23. The first phase of swallowing that is evaluated when the client has impaired swallowing is the _____ phase.

24. A 1 L bag of 5% dextrose in water IV solution contains only _____ kilocalories.

25. Ginger ale, apple juice, and gelatin are considered to be part of a _____ liquid diet.

26. A _____ gram sodium diet is common for clients with hypertension.

27. If a client has severe kidney disease, such as renal failure, protein is generally _____ in the diet.

EXERCISING YOUR CLINICAL JUDGMENT

Mrs. Goldman, the 54-year-old Russian woman introduced in the chapter case study, is receiving chemotherapy following surgery for breast cancer. Her nursing diagnosis is *Imbalanced nutrition: less than body requirements related to adverse effects of chemotherapy*. Specifically, she has early satiety and anorexia and says that food does not have much taste. You are working with Mrs. Goldman in the clinic setting to increase her nutritional intake with a Kosher diet, especially during the 3 remaining months of chemotherapy.

28. To increase Mrs. Goldman's sense of taste, you would recommend that she take supplemental doses of which of the following minerals?
    1. Magnesium
    2. Calcium
    3. Zinc
    4. Iodine

29. You would encourage Mrs. Goldman to increase intake at which of the following times, when intake is usually best?
    1. Breakfast
    2. Lunch
    3. Dinner
    4. Bedtime

30. To reduce the discomfort of mouth sores (xerostomia) that can accompany chemotherapy, you would advise Mrs. Goldman to avoid foods that have which of the following characteristics?
    1. Low in fat
    2. Spicy or acidic
    3. High in carbohydrates
    4. High in liquid content

31. To determine whether Mrs. Goldman has effectively increased the amount of iron in her diet, you would review the results of which of the following laboratory studies drawn at the next clinic visit?
    1. Blood urea nitrogen (BUN)
    2. Total protein
    3. Albumin
    4. Hemoglobin

TEST YOURSELF

32. The nurse giving enteral nutrition and medications through a feeding tube uses which of the following methods to prevent the tube from becoming occluded?
    1. Adequate flushing with water
    2. Instillation of meat tenderizer
    3. Flushing with cola
    4. Flushing with cranberry juice

33. The nurse measures and documents gastric residual for a client receiving enteral nutrition at which of the following time intervals?
    1. Hourly
    2. Every 2 hours
    3. Every 4 hours
    4. Every day

34. A client is receiving parenteral nutrition via a central venous catheter. The nurse monitors this client for fluid overload from hyperosmolar fluids most effectively by taking which of the following actions?
    1. Monitoring temperature
    2. Listening to lung sounds
    3. Checking results of serum osmolarity
    4. Watching the color of the urine

35. The nurse would interpret that a client has had a mild reaction to lipid emulsion infusion if the client experiences which of the following?
    1. Fever and chills
    2. Vomiting
    3. Pain in the back or chest
    4. Itchy skin rash

36. The nurse would best promote effective swallowing in a client at risk for aspiration by placing the client in which of the following positions?
    1. On the right side with the head elevated to 45 degrees
    2. Upright with the neck flexed at 45 degrees
    3. Supine and on the left side
    4. In a comfortable chair that promotes relaxation

Copyright © 2004, Elsevier Science (USA). All Rights Reserved.

Maintaining Fluid and Electrolyte Balance

PURPOSE

The purpose of this chapter is to introduce the concepts of fluid balance and its relationship to electrolytes in the body. You will learn introductory skills in providing intravenous therapy using physician orders.

MATCHING

1. ____ active transport
2. ____ anion
3. ____ cation
4. ____ colloid
5. ____ colloid osmotic pressure
6. ____ diffusion
7. ____ electrolyte
8. ____ filtration
9. ____ hydrostatic pressure
10. ____ hypotonic
11. ____ hypertonic
12. ____ isotonic
13. ____ metabolic acidosis
14. ____ metabolic alkalosis
15. ____ milliequivalent
16. ____ milliosmole
17. ____ nonelectrolyte
18. ____ osmolality
19. ____ osmolarity
20. ____ osmosis
21. ____ third spacing

a. a process in which molecules move from an area of lower concentration to an area of higher concentration through an expenditure of energy

b. a passive process by which molecules move through a cell membrane from an area of higher concentration to an area of lower concentration without an expenditure of energy

c. macromolecules that are too large to pass though a cell membrane and do not readily dissolve into a solution (e.g., protein)

d. the movement of water through a semipermeable membrane from an area containing a lesser concentration of particles to an area of greater concentration of particles

e. osmotic pressure exerted by the protein molecules

f. positively charged ion (e.g., sodium, potassium, calcium, magnesium, hydrogen)

g. the passage of water and certain smaller particles through a semipermeable membrane, assisted by hydrostatic or capillary pressure

h. substance that, when placed in a solvent such as water, breaks up into positively charged particles called ions; will conduct electricity

i. the number of milliosmoles per liter of solution

j. pressure exerted by the fluid within a compartment that results from the weight of the fluid; for practical purposes it can be thought of as the portion of the pressure exerted by the fluid itself

k. substance that does not ionize, thus does not carry an electrical charge (e.g., glucose)

l. the movement of fluid into an area in which the fluid is physiologically unavailable to the body (e.g., peritoneal space—ascites; pericardial

Copyright © 2004, Elsevier Science (USA). All Rights Reserved.

space—pericardial effusion; pleural space—pleural effusion; vesicles—burn)

m. the number of milliosmoles per kilogram of water

n. a pathological condition caused by an increase in bicarbonate or a decrease in acid, or both, in the extracellular fluid

o. a pathological condition caused by an increase in noncarbonic acids or a decrease in bicarbonate, or both, in the extracellular fluid

p. the unit of force from the dissolved particles in a solution

q. having an osmotic pressure less than that of the solution with which it is being compared

r. one thousandth of a chemical equivalent; the measurement used to express the chemical activity or combining power of an ion

s. having an osmotic pressure equal to that of the solution with which it is being compared

t. having an osmotic pressure greater than that of the solution with which it is being compared

u. negatively charged ion (e.g., chloride, bicarbonate, phosphate, sulfate, proteinate)

TRUE OR FALSE

22. ____ Clients with hyponatremia should be observed for low urinary output.

23. ____ Clients with hypernatremia should be observed for fluid retention.

24. ____ The most characteristic manifestations of hypokalemia are muscle flaccidity and ECG changes.

25. ____ Hyperkalemia occurs in the presence of high volume urinary output.

26. ____ The client with hypocalcemia should be observed for seizures.

27. ____ Hypercalcemia is associated with kidney stones.

28. ____ Insensible water loss should be measured as part of intake and output.

29. ____ Cardiac failure is associated with retention of potassium and water.

30. ____ Tube feedings are hypertonic, thus the client may be at risk for fluid volume deficit unless water is given as a supplement.

31. ____ 5% Dextrose in water is given primarily for its glucose content.

32. ____ 5% Dextrose in 1/2 normal saline (a 25% solution) given at 3000 cc per day does not add sodium to the body.

33. ____ Hyponatremia can result from administration of excess D_5W.

34. ____ Plasma is used as a volume expander when a client is bleeding and there is not time to type and cross-match blood.

35. ____ Caution should be used with IV therapy to prevent air from entering a client's veins.

FILL-IN-THE-BLANKS

36. Glucocorticoids cause _____ (retention, excretion) of fluid.

37. To pass a nasogastric tube you should use a _____-_____ lubricant.

38. Nasogastric suction is used for gastrointestinal _____ in the presence of a bowel _____.

39. In a burn client fluid is lost by _____ _____.

40. To pass a nasogastric tube, the client should be in the _____ _____ position.

41. _____ _____ is the only acceptable irrigant for a nasogastric tube.

42. When selecting an IV site you should start with the most _____ (distal, proximal) vein that would support an intravenous catheter.

43. A(n) _____ -gauge needle is used for a venipuncture if you have reason to believe the client may need blood.

44. To clean a site for venipuncture, start _____ _____ _____ and clean in a circular motion _____ _____ (toward, away from) the site.

45. When you make a venipuncture, you confirm that you are in the vein by observing _____ _____.

EXERCISING YOUR CLINICAL JUDGMENT

Mrs. Thompson, the woman introduced in this chapter's case study, has experienced two types of fluid imbalance within the past few weeks. She is currently admitted to the hospital with congestive heart failure resulting from excess fluid volume.

46. Which of the following signs of excess fluid volume would the admitting nurse expect to note in Mrs. Thompson at the time of admission to the hospital?
    1. A weak thready pulse
    2. Sluggish skin turgor
    3. Neck vein distention
    4. Postural hypotension

47. Which of the following electrolyte values could be expected to accompany Mrs. Thompson's fluid volume excess?
    1. Sodium 131 mEq/L
    2. Potassium 5.4 mEq/L
    3. Sodium 140 mEq/L
    4. Potassium 4.3 mEq/L

48. Which of the following basic nursing interventions focused on fluid volume excess should be included in a care plan for Mrs. Thompson?
    1. Assess breath sounds.
    2. Assess the diet for potassium content.
    3. Encourage increased fluid intake.
    4. Discourage use of salt substitutes.

49. Mrs. Thompson has an order for 500 ml 0.9% sodium chloride to run at a keep vein open rate of 20 ml/hr. An infusion pump is not available. After selecting a microdrip infusion set with a calibration of 60 drops/ml, you would adjust the IV to deliver how many drops per minute (gtt/min) of solution?
    1. 10
    2. 20
    3. 30
    4. 33

50. Which of the following assessments provides the best evaluative data that Mrs. Thompson's fluid balance is returning to normal?
    1. Heart rate is 100 beats per minute
    2. Voided 500 ml the previous 8-hour shift
    3. Weight has returned to baseline
    4. Took in 360 ml with breakfast

TEST YOURSELF

51. Six hours postsurgery your client has signs of deficient fluid volume. The doctor orders a fluid challenge of 200 cc lactated Ringer's intravenously over 20 minutes stat. You should assess for a positive response to this treatment by observing for which of the following?
    1. Decrease in blood pressure
    2. Crackles in lower lung bases
    3. Increase in specific gravity
    4. Increase in renal output

52. Prior to administering a potassium supplement it is most important that the nurse assess the function of which of the following body systems?
    1. Hepatic
    2. Cerebral
    3. Renal
    4. Vascular

53. You determine that your client has been taking his diuretic at home whenever he thinks he needs it. Which of the following would be a typical side effect of excess furosemide (Lasix) to monitor for during visits to the health center?
    1. Nephrosis
    2. Metabolic acidosis
    3. Hypokalemia
    4. Hypernatremia

54. The nursing care plan for hypovolemia should include which of the following?
    1. Increasing fluid intake to 2000cc/day
    2. Placing client in the supine position
    3. Increasing protein in the client's diet
    4. Auscultating for adventitious breath sounds

55. The most accurate means of determining the amount of fluid retention in an individual is by which of the following means?
    1. Measuring edema with a millimeter tape
    2. Accurately measuring the client's intake
    3. Determining the amount of neck vein distention
    4. Classifying edema as 1+, 2+, 3+, or 4+

56. Which one of the following vitamins plays the most important role in calcium absorption in the presence of hypocalcemia?
    1. Vitamin A
    2. Vitamin D
    3. Vitamin B
    4. Vitamin E

57. A 45-year-old client has just returned to your unit after major abdominal surgery. Based on the impact of antidiuretic hormone (ADH) released during the stress of surgery, select the most likely client response.
    1. Increased urinary output for the first 24 hours
    2. Decreased urinary output for the first 24 hours
    3. No change in output from the previous 24 hours
    4. Intake equal to output for the first 24 hours

58. Signs and symptoms of circulatory overload include which of the following?
    1. Cold, clammy skin; decreased BP; SOB; hacking cough
    2. Rales, moist cough, neck vein distention, increased BP
    3. Decreased venous pressure, cyanosis, SOB, orthopnea
    4. Decreased BP; pitting edema; cold, dry skin

59. While reviewing your patient's lab test you note a seriously low serum calcium. Which of the following would be an appropriate nursing intervention to incorporate into your care?
    1. Force fluid to 12 glasses per day.
    2. Monitor intake and output.
    3. Provide a quiet nonstimulating environment.
    4. Encourage bananas and orange juice in the diet.

60. Your client is to receive an intravenous infusion of 1000 D_5W over 10 hours. Your drip chamber delivers 15 gtts/1 cc. How many drops per minute would you run the IV infusion?
    1. 33
    2. 25
    3. 20
    4. 16

Promoting Wound Healing

PURPOSE

This chapter discusses key concepts that relate to the nursing diagnoses *Risk for impaired skin integrity, Impaired skin integrity,* and *Impaired tissue integrity*. It describes the skin disruptions, wound health, and problems of wound healing.

MATCHING

1. ____ abrasion

2. ____ debridement

3. ____ dehiscence

4. ____ epithelialization

5. ____ eschar

6. ____ evisceration

7. ____ exudate

8. ____ fistula

9. ____ hematoma

10. ____ hemorrhage

11. ____ laceration

12. ____ pressure ulcer

13. ____ primary lesion

14. ____ secondary lesion

15. ____ wound

a. a disruption of normal anatomic structure and function that results from bodily injury or a pathological process that may begin internally or externally to the involved organ or organs

b. thick, leathery, necrotic, devitalized tissue

c. refers to the fluid and cells that have escaped from blood vessels during the inflammatory response and are left in the surrounding tissues

d. an accumulation of bloody fluid beneath tissue

e. the first lesion to appear on the skin in response to a causative agent

f. a superficial injury caused by rubbing or scraping the skin against another surface

g. bleeding from the wound bed or site

h. an abnormal passage between two internal organs or between an organ and the external skin surface

i. refers to a partial or total separation of the wound edges

j. the protrusion of an internal organ (such as a bowel loop) through the incision

k. the removal of dirt, foreign matter, and dead or devitalized tissue from a wound

l. a process in which epithelial cells move to the wound bed

m. open wound with jagged edges

n. any lesion caused by unrelieved pressure that leads to damage of underlying tissues

o. a lesion that results when changes occur in a primary lesion

TRUE OR FALSE

16. ____ Skin lesions are related to the client's medical condition.

17. ____ A black wound indicates that the wound is not yet ready to heal because it has fibrous slough or exudate that must be cleansed and removed.

18. ____ Most acute wounds and surgical wounds close by primary intention.

19. ____ Internal hemorrhage can occur with no external evidence of bleeding.

20. ____ Wounds can heal when infection is present.

21. ____ Yellow drainage from a wound means the wound is infected.

Copyright © 2004, Elsevier Science (USA). All Rights Reserved.

22. ____ Radiation is the least common mechanism of skin injury.

FILL-IN-THE-BLANKS

23. _____ is the primary function of the skin.

24. The _____-_____-_____ (RYB) classification system is based on wound bed color.

25. Typically, a _____ _____ is located over a bony prominence or an area that sustains prolonged pressure.

26. The single most important factor in preventing wound infections and promoting wound healing is strict _____ and _____ asepsis.

27. Use the concept of the face of a _____ to help define landmarks and areas of the wound or impaired skin area.

28. Surgical wounds and incisions are usually closed with _____ or stainless steel _____.

29. Interventions for a client with *Impaired skin integrity* are developed by the multidisciplinary team. A valuable resource to medical and nursing staff is the certified _____ therapist nurse.

EXERCISING YOUR CLINICAL JUDGMENT

30. Mrs. Jacan, the client from the chapter's case study, is bedridden after her hip surgery. She has developed a pressure ulcer that looks like a blister or shallow crater. Her pressure ulcer is most likely in which stage?
    1. Stage I
    2. Stage II
    3. Stage III
    4. Stage IV

31. Mrs. Jacan is given which one of the following diagnostic tests to help determine if she has inflammation, infectious, or necrotic processes?
    a. Complete blood count
    2. Erythrocyte sedimentation rate
    3. Prealbumin and albumin levels
    4. Blood panel

32. Mrs. Jacan had a reddened area on her sacrum and bilateral heels. Twenty-four hours after admission, you chart the following: Hydrocolloid dressing intact, no drainage (you had applied dressings to her sacrum and to her heels). Which of the following nursing diagnoses would be most appropriate for your evaluation of your client's care?
    1. *Impaired tissue integrity*
    2. *Disturbed body image*
    3. *Hopelessness*
    4. *Impaired skin integrity*

TEST YOURSELF

33. Your client was wounded by a knife. What type of wound is your client most likely suffering from?
    1. Closed and clean wound
    2. Abrasion and contusion
    3. Open, contaminated, penetrating
    4. Open, contaminated, abrasion

34. The area around your client's wound has edema, erythema, heat, and pain. His wound is 1 day old. This is an example of which phase of wound healing?
    1. Inflammatory
    2. Proliferative
    3. Reconstruction
    4. Maturation

35. If your client has an incision and dressing on the anterior part of the neck, you would check which of the following to determine if she was hemorrhaging externally?
    1. Bloody drainage on dressing, distention of the affected area, a change in the amount or type of drainage from a drain
    2. Distention of the affected area, a change in the amount or type of drainage from a drain, signs and symptoms of hypovolemic shock
    3. Bloody drainage on dressing, signs and symptoms of hypovolemic shock
    4. Bloody drainage on dressing and areas around the dressing and posterior to the wound site

36. Your client is a single 38-year-old female on her third postoperative day. She is very concerned about the large abdominal incision created during her hysterectomy and worries how this will affect her relationship with men she dates. Which of the following nursing diagnoses would be most appropriate?
    1. *Impaired tissue integrity*
    2. *Disturbed body image*
    3. *Hopelessness*
    4. *Impaired skin integrity*

37. For a wound to heal, the wound must be clean and free of bacteria. To cleanse a wound, you will need a wound cleaning solution. Which of the following is the preferred cleansing agent for most wounds?
    1. Normal saline solution
    2. Dakin's solution
    3. Povidone-iodine
    4. Hydrogen peroxide

Copyright © 2004, Elsevier Science (USA). All Rights Reserved.

Managing Body Temperature

27

PURPOSE

The purpose of this chapter is to introduce you to the concepts of thermoregulation and associated clinical problems.

MATCHING

1. ____ fever
2. ____ heat exhaustion
3. ____ heatstroke
4. ____ hyperthermia
5. ____ hypothermia
6. ____ malaise
7. ____ pyrogen
8. ____ set-point

a. a nonregulated elevation in body temperature related to an imbalance between heat gain and heat loss

b. the temperature that thermoregulatory mechanisms attempt to maintain

c. the body temperature exceeds 40.6° C (105° F), resulting in altered central nervous system function and shock

d. a feeling of indisposition; is thought to be an adaptive response that decreases most daily activities, thereby maintaining energy stores for fever generation

e. any agent that causes or stimulates a fever; the initial stimulus for fever is often exogenous pyrogen

f. a regulated rise in body temperature that is mediated by a rise in temperature set-point

g. state in which body temperature is reduced below normal

h. a rise in body temperature that is usually related to inadequate fluid and electrolyte replacement during physical activity in intense heat or the inability to acclimatize to intense heat

TRUE OR FALSE

9. ____ Fever is caused only by infection.

10. ____ During the initiation phase of a fever, pyrogens act on the hypothalamus to reset the temperature set-point higher than body temperature.

11. ____ Resolution of a fever by lysis is a gradual return to normal over several hours.

12. ____ Determination of the cause of fever can be difficult because of the many possible etiologies.

13. ____ A common finding in hypothermic clients is the incidence of low alcohol or other drug intake

14. ____ An immunosuppressed client is able to generate a fever.

15. ____ Fever may not develop as readily in the elderly as in the younger population.

16. ____ Treatment for arthritis may mask a fever.

17. ____ Blood cultures are only used to identify bacteria in the blood.

18. ____ Blood cultures are best drawn through a central line IV site.

19. ____ An elderly client is more prone to heatstroke than a young adult.

20. ____ Febrile convulsions in infants are associated with temperatures greater than 105° F.

21. ____ Vasoconstriction decreases heat loss by radiation, convection, and conduction.

22. ____ In some clients, fever may not be present during infection.

23. ____ Hyperthermia occurs when a person falls through the ice of a lake and loses heat rapidly in the cold water.

24. ____ The change in heart rate with hypothermia will depend on the degree of hypothermia.

25. ____ The height of a child's fever does not seem to trigger febrile convulsions as much as a sudden spike in body temperature.

Copyright © 2004, Elsevier Science (USA). All Rights Reserved.

FILL-IN-THE-BLANKS

26. The three phases of a fever are _____, _____, and _____.

27. During fever the metabolic rate increases by _____ for every degree of increase in temperature.

28. A client with a fever has a(n) _____ (increased, decreased) need for fluids.

29. The symptoms of heatstroke include _____ _____, _____, _____, _____, and _____.

30. Alcohol use contributes to hypothermia by providing a false sense of _____, inhibiting _____ and _____ of the skin.

31. _____ _____ or fever of unknown origin is defined as fever of 3 weeks' duration with evaluation by a medical team for 1 week.

32. Side effects of aspirin include _____ and _____.

33. Acetaminophen should not be used in the presence of _____ disease.

34. Cooling blankets promote _____ heat loss.

35. Fans promote _____ heat loss.

36. Physical cooling is the standard for _____ (hyperthermia, fever).

37. _____ is the resolution of a fever.

38. The temperature control center is in the _____.

39. The two classes of interventions used for treating fever include _____ and _____ _____.

40. To assess for tolerance before feeding a febrile client you would assess for _____ _____, _____ _____, and _____.

EXERCISING YOUR CLINICAL JUDGMENT

41. Mr. Stephen is 24 hours' post cardiac bypass surgical procedure. His temperature is 102° F. You find signs of postoperative atelectasis and encourage him to cough and deep breathe. How often should you recheck his temperature?
    1. q4h
    2. qid
    3. bid
    4. q8h

42. A physician has written an order for Mr. Stephen for acetaminophen for a temperature greater than 102° F. A rationale for not giving the antipyretic for a lower temperature is that:
    1. fever is a host defense response.
    2. normal temperature is variable.
    3. antipyretics only work on high temperatures.
    4. only a high fever produces a headache.

TEST YOURSELF

43. A mother of a 3-year-old asks for your advice about which antipyretic to use for her child's fever. Your best response would be:
    1. "Use acetaminophen. It is the best antipyretic."
    2. "Pediatricians often recommend avoiding aspirin in young children."
    3. "Never give your child antipyretics without the advice of a physician."
    4. "Acetaminophen can cause Reye's syndrome in young children."

44. A mother calls the emergency room. Her 6-year-old child has a fever of 101° F. Which information that she provides would prompt you to refer her to a physician?
    1. The child has not been exposed to a contagious disease.
    2. The child is having difficulty breathing.
    3. The child has clear drainage from the nose.
    4. The child is constipated.

45. A client with osteoarthritis has a painful swollen knee joint. Her temperature is 99.6° F. Select the best interpretation of her fever.
    1. Her knee has become infected.
    2. Her temperature is normally high.
    3. Her temperature is caused by inflammation.
    4. She is having a reaction to her medication.

46. Heatstroke results from:
    1. failure of the temperature-regulating capacity of the body, caused by prolonged exposure to the sun.
    2. a rupture of a blood vessel in the brain from getting overheated.
    3. pyrogens building up in the bloodstream because of kidney failure.
    4. a bacterial infection that attacks the temperature control center of the brain.

Copyright © 2004, Elsevier Science (USA). All Rights Reserved.

Managing Bowel Elimination

PURPOSE

This chapter introduces you to alterations in bowel elimination such as constipation, diarrhea, and bowel incontinence. It describes a variety of factors that affect bowel function and discusses the nursing process as a framework to use when caring for a client with an alteration in bowel elimination.

MATCHING

1. ____ bowel incontinence
2. ____ cathartic
3. ____ colostomy
4. ____ constipation
5. ____ diarrhea
6. ____ fecal impaction
7. ____ feces
8. ____ flatus
9. ____ flatulence
10. ____ guaiac
11. ____ ileostomy
12. ____ laxative
13. ____ occult blood
14. ____ ostomy
15. ____ paralytic ileus
16. ____ peristalsis
17. ____ steatorrhea
18. ____ stoma

a. the rhythmic smooth muscle contractions of the intestinal wall that propel the intestinal contents forward

b. body waste discharged from the intestine

c. the presence of abnormal amounts of gas in the GI tract, causing abdominal distention and discomfort

d. an amount of blood that is too small to be seen without a microscope

e. an amount of gas that occurs normally in the GI tract

f. the inability to voluntarily control the passage of feces and gas

g. a surgical procedure involving the creation of an opening between the colon and the abdominal wall

h. medication used to induce emptying of the bowel; often used interchangeably with a laxative, although it has a stronger action

i. a condition in which feces are abnormally hard and dry and evacuation is abnormally infrequent

j. a gray stool mixed with observable fat and mucus, resulting from the malabsorption of fat

k. the opening between the abdominal wall and intestine through which fecal material passes

l. the surgical procedure used to create an opening through the abdominal wall and into the intestine

m. the absence of peristalsis for more than 3 days

n. a test to measure occult blood

o. a collection of puttylike or hardened feces in the rectum or sigmoid colon that prevents the passage of a normal stool and becomes more hardened as the colon continues to absorb water from it

p. medication used to induce emptying of the bowel; often used interchangeably with cathartic

q. a surgical procedure involving the creation of an opening between the ileum and the abdominal wall

r. the rapid movement of fecal matter through the intestine, resulting in poor absorption of water, nutrients, and electrolytes, and producing abnormally frequent evacuation of watery stools

Copyright © 2004, Elsevier Science (USA). All Rights Reserved.

TRUE OR FALSE

19. ____ Constipation is a major complaint among the elderly.

20. ____ Some risks of straining at stool include angina attacks, hemorrhoid development, and rupture of abdominal suture lines.

21. ____ It is exceptionally difficult to train the bowel to evacuate at a certain time.

22. ____ Spicy foods stimulate peristalsis by local reflex stimulation.

23. ____ Exercise has no effect on bowel elimination.

24. ____ Bowel elimination is usually not a problem for the adolescent unless there is a health problem.

25. ____ Motor or sensory disturbances, such as with spinal cord injury or neurological disease, can lead to diarrhea.

26. ____ A medication that is given to prevent constipation can cause diarrhea in some clients.

27. ____ The further down the bowel a colostomy is created, the greater the chance for being able to regulate the bowel.

28. ____ Mental depression plays no role in the development of constipation.

FILL-IN-THE-BLANKS

29. A diet that is high in _____ tends to prevent the occurrence of constipation.

30. Chocolate, coffee, and prune juice are foods that can _____ the stool.

31. _____ is an out-pouching of the intestinal wall that can occur after age 40.

32. Impaired dentition in the older adult impairs _____, allowing food to enter the GI tract inadequately chewed.

33. A client is more at risk for cancer of the colon if the diet is high in _____ and low in _____.

34. The consistency of ileostomy drainage is _____.

35. As part of colon cancer screening, an annual digital rectal examination should be done every year after age _____.

36. Beans, beer, and cucumbers are examples of foods that can cause _____.

37. How the GI tract reacts to a particular food depends on the individual _____.

38. The overuse of laxatives can lead to physical and psychological _____.

EXERCISING YOUR CLINICAL JUDGMENT

Dr. Daley, the 92-year-old retired neurosurgeon introduced in the chapter case study, has a nursing diagnosis of *Constipation*. He is living in a long-term care facility because he can no longer manage on his own with a diagnosis of bone cancer. He has begun limiting the use of his opioid analgesic, morphine, because it could worsen the constipation. The nurse from the previous shift reports having just assessed Dr. Daley's abdomen and suspects impaction. You are now taking over the care of the clients on this unit.

39. Dr. Daley has chosen to use Milk of Magnesia as his laxative. You recall that this medication belongs to which of the following categories of laxatives?
    1. Bulk-forming
    2. Lubricant
    3. Saline
    4. Stimulant

40. The medication given to Dr. Daley has not worked, so you obtain an order for an oil retention enema. When administering it to Dr. Daley, you ask him to try to retain it in the bowel for at least how long?
    1. 5 minutes
    2. 15 minutes
    3. 30 minutes
    4. An hour

41. The enema is successful and you are exploring with Dr. Daley strategies that can be used to prevent a recurrence. You both agree that he should try to walk to the toilet at which of the following times, when stimulation of the gastrocolic reflex is strongest?
    1. Upon awakening
    2. After breakfast
    3. After lunch
    4. Before bedtime

42. You begin an intake and output record to keep track of Dr. Daley's fluid intake. You encourage him to drink at least how much fluid per day to minimize the risk of constipation recurrence?
    1. 1.5 liters
    2. 3 liters
    3. 4 liters
    4. 5 liters

Copyright © 2004, Elsevier Science (USA). All Rights Reserved.

TEST YOURSELF

43. The nurse caring for a client with an ostomy would do which of the following to maintain the skin integrity around the stoma?
    1. Use a skin barrier.
    2. Limit the use of skin paste.
    3. Wash peristomal skin but do not dry it.
    4. Try to have the pouch last about 2 weeks.

44. A client has abdominal pain related to flatulence. Which of the following items would the nurse suspect is contributing to the problem?
    1. Walking
    2. Eating slowly
    3. Eating cauliflower
    4. Drinking water

45. The nurse changing a client's ostomy bag should cut a new appliance how much larger than the size of the client's stoma to have a proper fit?
    1. 1/16 inch
    2. 1/8 inch
    3. 1/4 inch
    4. 1/2 inch

46. A client with diarrhea was treated with antibiotic therapy and now would benefit from recolonization of normal GI flora. The nurse should offer this client which of the following products?
    1. Cheese
    2. Yogurt
    3. Skim milk
    4. Raw apples

47. An older adult with multiple health problems has a severe case of diarrhea. The nurse would assess this client for which of the following common complications of diarrhea in this client population?
    1. Thirst and ruddy skin color
    2. Diverticulitis
    3. Nausea and vomiting
    4. Fluid and electrolyte imbalances

Copyright © 2004, Elsevier Science (USA). All Rights Reserved.

Managing Urinary Elimination

PURPOSE

This chapter introduces you to basic nursing measures for clients with urinary problems. You will learn to recognize signs and symptoms of urinary problems and intervene to improve urinary function. Additionally, the chapter introduces procedures for collecting a urine specimen from a Foley catheter, using a condom catheter, and inserting a Foley catheter.

MATCHING

1. ____ anuria

2. ____ bacteriuria

3. ____ diuresis

4. ____ dysuria

5. ____ enuresis

6. ____ hematuria

7. ____ Kegel exercises

8. ____ micturition

9. ____ nocturia

10. ____ oliguria

11. ____ polyuria

12. ____ reflex incontinence

13. ____ residual urine

14. ____ stress incontinence

15. ____ total incontinence

16. ____ urge incontinence

17. ____ urinalysis

18. ____ urinary frequency

19. ____ urinary hesitancy

20. ____ urinary incontinence

21. ____ urinary retention

22. ____ urinary urgency

23. ____ urination

a. recurrent involuntary urination that occurs during sleep

b. the term used for nighttime urination

c. involuntary passage of urine

d. the person is unaware of cues to a full bladder and may be unaware of the incontinence; the incontinence is either continual or unpredictable

e. incontinence associated with neurological damage to the spinal cord above the level of the third sacral vertebrae

f. the inability to pass all or part of the urine that has accumulated in the bladder

g. incontinence reported or observed as dribbling with increased intra-abdominal pressure

h. the discharge of blood in the urine

i. incontinence reported or observed as a sudden desire to urinate and immediately seeking toileting facilities

j. the more commonly used term for the act of micturition; the term *void* is more common in clinical use

k. the increased secretion of urine

l. the symptom of difficulty with, or painful, urination; it may be accompanied by frequency, hesitancy, or urgency of urination

m. the absence of urine production

n. the amount of urine remaining in the bladder after voiding

o. sudden, forceful urge to urinate; further assessment is needed to determine the cause

p. a physical, chemical, and microscopic examination of the urine

q. urination that occurs at shorter-than-usual intervals without an increase in daily urine output

r. a diminished, scanty amount of urine

s. a large amount of urine usually associated with diabetes mellitus or diabetes insipidus

t. exercises to strengthen the floor of the pelvis

u. bacteria in the urine

v. the process of emptying the bladder

w. a delay in starting the urine stream, commonly with a decreased force of stream

TRUE OR FALSE

24. ____ The bladder is under the involuntary control of the sympathetic nervous system.

25. ____ Enuresis occurs by the age of 8 years in all but about 7% of children.

26. ____ Urinary retention can be caused by obstruction or inability of the detrusor to contract.

27. ____ Urinary incontinence is an expected or normal part of aging.

28. ____ Six to eight glasses of water is equivalent to 1500 to 2000 ml.

29. ____ The external urinary sphincter is smooth muscle under control of the parasympathetic nervous system.

30. ____ A primary factor in incontinence for some elderly persons is urge incontinence in the presence of impaired mobility.

31. ____ Constipation can be a factor in incontinence of urine.

32. ____ Bilirubin is excreted in the urine when the biliary tract is obstructed.

33. ____ There is no reason to test the urine for blood unless the urine is red or cloudy.

34. ____ You need a minimum of 30 ml of urine to send for urinalysis.

35. ____ All clients need an antibiotic after a cystoscopy.

FILL-IN-THE-BLANKS

36. The _____ valve is the connection between the ureters and the bladder.

37. The _____ is the primary muscle of the bladder.

38. The kidneys control the excretion of these waste products: _____, _____, _____ _____, _____, and _____ _____ _____.

39. Among other electrolytes, the kidneys control the excretion of the two primary electrolytes, _____ and _____.

40. Urine moves through the ureters by gravity and _____.

41. Dysuria is often related to _____, _____, or _____ of the lower urinary tract.

42. Voiding every hour would be described as _____.

43. The normal range for feeling the urge to urinate is _____ to _____ ml.

44. _____ _____ measures the function of the bladder and urethra by measuring the flow rate of urine passing through the urethra.

45. _____ (creatinine, BUN) is the more specific test for renal function.

46. _____ incontinence is associated with postmenopausal atrophy or the presence of a cystocele.

47. The Alzheimer's client who has progressed to the point of no neurological control over the bladder has _____ or _____ incontinence.

48. As a means to control incontinence _____ _____ is recommended for clients who can learn to recognize some degree of bladder fullness or the need to void.

49. As a means to control incontinence _____ _____ is recommended for clients for whom a natural pattern of voiding can be determined.

50. _____ _____ can help the client who has stress incontinence.

EXERCISING YOUR CLINICAL JUDGMENT

Fatima Shireem, the case study client introduced in this chapter, is scheduled to have an indwelling urinary catheter removed this morning. It is now her second postoperative day following vaginal hysterectomy surgery. You have been assigned to Mrs. Shireem's care for the day shift.

Copyright © 2004, Elsevier Science (USA). All Rights Reserved.

51. For what reason is it most important that Mrs. Shireem's catheter be removed as early as possible in the course of recovery from surgery?
    1. Because of the high risk of infection
    2. Because she has a higher risk of retention with each passing day
    3. Because an indwelling catheter often provokes bladder spasms
    4. Because she will ambulate more easily without the catheter and drainage bag

52. To minimize discomfort during the removal of the catheter, you should ask Mrs. Shireem to do which of the following during catheter removal?
    1. Cough
    2. Take a deep breath
    3. Bear down as if to void
    4. Encourage her to squeeze your hand

53. The catheter was removed at 8:30 AM. On the report sheet to be used later in the day for intershift report, you note that Mrs. Shireem is due to void *no later than* which of the following times?
    1. 10:30 AM
    2. 2:30 PM
    3. 4:30 PM
    4. 8:30 PM

54. Which of the following instructions would be best to give to Mrs. Shireem to increase the likelihood that she will void successfully after catheter removal?
    1. Ambulate at least hourly
    2. Take a diet of clear liquids only
    3. Encourage her to keep a bedpan nearby
    4. Encourage her to increase her fluid intake

TEST YOURSELF

55. You are assessing a 57-year-old female client. She says she continues to have stress incontinence despite using the Kegel exercises regularly for 6 months. Her doctor has talked about surgery, but she is reluctant. She asks you if she should keep trying the exercises. Which of the following is the best response?
    1. "If you haven't had success in 6 months, you should see your doctor about surgery."
    2. "I can review the technique with you if you like; sometimes it is difficult to contract the right muscle."
    3. "Kegel exercises only work for a small number of women."
    4. "It is always best to follow your doctor's advice."

56. Which of the following techniques is best to prevent the most serious complication of a condom catheter?
    1. To hold the catheter in place, use a soft flexible band that is snug but not tight.
    2. Inspect and clean the skin at least daily.
    3. Arrange the drainage tubing to ensure urine drains from the condom.
    4. Tape the catheter collecting tubing to the leg, allowing slack in the catheter.

57. You are assigned a client who has urinary incontinence. You see a nursing order on the care plan for prompted voiding. To correctly assist with this intervention you would take which of the following actions?
    1. Take the client to the bathroom every 4 hours or offer the bedpan.
    2. Insist that the client go to the bathroom or use the bedpan every 2 hours.
    3. Admonish the client for wetness and insist that the client use the call light.
    4. Check the client for wetness every 2 hours and offer assistance to the bathroom or bedside commode.

58. Which of the following clients is the best candidate for whom a Foley catheter may be used to prevent urinary retention?
    1. A client who has had bladder surgery where some bleeding is expected
    2. A client who has had surgery for a fractured hip
    3. A client who is in shock (blood pressure 88/50)
    4. A client with terminal cancer, who is expected to die within 24 hours

59. Your client is a 60-year-old male. He is 6' 4" tall and weighs 225 pounds. Select the catheter size that is most likely to be appropriate.
    1. 10 Fr
    2. 14 Fr
    3. 16 Fr
    4. 18 Fr

60. You are performing a Foley catheterization. You accidentally contaminate the connection tubing, but know the catheter is sterile. Which of the following actions would be most cost effective and still be correct?
    1. Ask someone to bring you a new sterile catheter.
    2. Obtain a new tray and start over.
    3. Ask someone to bring you a new sterile bag and tubing.
    4. Continue with the catheterization, avoiding the connection tubing until you have inserted the catheter.

Copyright © 2004, Elsevier Science (USA). All Rights Reserved.

61. Which of the following is the best rationale for maintaining straight continuous gravity drainage from a Foley catheter?
    1. To be more aesthetically pleasing to the client
    2. To prevent the backflow of urine into the bladder
    3. To keep the bladder empty of urine
    4. To keep the catheter patent

62. Your client has had bladder surgery. The surgeon has ordered a three-way Foley with continuous irrigation with normal saline. You enter the room and notice that the urine is dark red with only a small amount flowing through the drainage tubing. Which of the following is the best action to take?
    1. Call the surgeon immediately.
    2. Force fluids by mouth.
    3. Increase the flow of the irrigant until the urine clears.
    4. Turn the client in bed.

63. Your client has a urinary diversion that is well healed and has been functioning normally. She is currently admitted for pneumonia, is very weak, and needs assistance with caring for her elimination needs. You notice that urine is leaking under the stoma wafer applied to her skin. Which of the following is the best action to take?
    1. Use nonporous tape to secure the wafer.
    2. Remove the wafer and apply a new one.
    3. Pad the site to collect the leakage.
    4. Remove the wafer and insert a catheter to collect the urine.

64. Which of the following suggestions to acidify the urine would be best to make to a client?
    1. Take 500 mg vitamin C BID.
    2. Drink four glasses of diluted cranberry juice daily.
    3. Use 1 teaspoon sodium bicarbonate BID.
    4. Drink four glasses of orange juice daily.

Copyright © 2004, Elsevier Science (USA). All Rights Reserved.

Managing Self-Care Deficit

PURPOSE

This chapter introduces you to key concepts that relate to the nursing diagnoses *Bathing/hygiene self-care deficit, Impaired skin integrity, Altered oral mucous membrane, Ineffective individual coping*, and *Powerlessness*. The chapter also outlines procedures related to assisting the client with self-care needs.

MATCHING

1. ____ alopecia

2. ____ caries

3. ____ cerumen

4. ____ dentures

5. ____ gingivitis

6. ____ perineum

7. ____ plaque

8. ____ tartar

a. a waxy secretion of the glands of the external acoustic meatus; it is commonly called earwax

b. a destructive process causing decalcification of the tooth enamel and leading to continued destruction of the enamel and dentin with resulting cavitation of the tooth

c. an inflammation of the gums usually manifested by the primary symptom of bleeding of the gums

d. a yellowish film of calcium phosphate, carbonate, food particles, and other organic matter deposited on the teeth by saliva

e. a complement of teeth, either natural or artificial, ordinarily used to designate an artificial replacement for the natural teeth

f. loss of hair and baldness

g. the pelvic floor and associated structures occupying pelvic outlet, bounded anteriorly by the symphysis pubis, laterally by the ischial tuberosities, and posteriorly by the coccyx

h. a soft, thin film of food debris, mucin and dead epithelial cells that is deposited on the teeth and provides a medium for the growth of bacteria

TRUE OR FALSE

9. ____ The outer portion of the skin, the epidermis, is composed of stratified squamous epithelium that contains keratinocytes, which produce keratin, the substance that is responsible for the color of the skin.

10. ____ Hair grows faster at night than during the day and faster in warm weather than in cold.

11. ____ If your nails are thick and yellow, this may be indicative of bacterial infection.

12. ____ If you presuppose lack of ability when some ability may be present it can further reinforce a client's sense of independence and helplessness.

13. ____ Total hygiene care consists of bathing, skin care, oral care, hair care, perineal care, back massage, shaving, changing the bed linens and changing a client's gown or pajamas.

14. ____ Problems with nail and foot care usually occur because of neglect or abuse.

15. ____ The benefits of bathing in a tub or shower (instead of a sponge bath) for the client are so significant that if the option is available, you should use it even if it may be difficult and time consuming.

16. ____ Studies show that a client who needs to be fed will eat more food if the person doing the feeding switches from one food to another during the meal.

Copyright © 2004, Elsevier Science (USA). All Rights Reserved.

FILL-IN-THE-BLANKS

17. _____ -_____ is the ability to meet hygiene needs without the assistance of another person.

18. The skin helps screen out ultraviolet (UV) rays from the sun, but it also lets in some necessary UV rays that convert a chemical in the skin called 7-dehydrocholesterol into _____.

19. If the origin of a client's halitosis is _____, oral hygiene will not remove the odor.

20. Dental _____ is a disease of the calcified structure of the tooth.

21. Body lice suck _____ from the skin and live in clothing, making them hard to detect.

22. Skin _____ are prominent in aging skin.

23. Complete _____ _____ is giving the complete bath without any assistance from the client.

24. For clients with very curly hair, it is often useful to use a _____-_____ comb or a hair _____.

EXERCISING YOUR CLINICAL JUDGMENT

25. Joy Wilson, the 78-year-old African-American client from the chapter's case study, suffers from a stroke (cerebrovascular accident). She is unable to bathe herself. Which nursing diagnosis would be most appropriate?
   1. *Ineffective individual coping*
   2. *Bathing/hygiene self-care deficit*
   3. *Activity intolerance*
   4. *Impaired physical mobility*

26. Ms. Wilson's daughter gives her a hot-water bath. Which of the following best describes the purpose of this type of bath?
   1. Decrease pain and inflammation
   2. Relieve muscle spasm and muscle tension
   3. Relax and soothe
   4. Soothe skin irritation

27. Ms. Wilson's cognitive status is impaired because of her short-term memory loss. She has difficulty caring for her basic needs. Which nursing diagnosis would be most appropriate?
   1. *Ineffective individual coping*
   2. *Bathing/hygiene self-care deficit*
   3. *Activity intolerance*
   4. *Disturbed thought processes*

TEST YOURSELF

28. You advise the client to do regular oral care and that dental intervention may be necessary. Which problem of the oral cavity is your client most likely suffering from?
   1. Halitosis
   2. Gingivitis
   3. Periodontal disease
   4. Stomatitis

29. Your client is having difficulty following through on doing self-care. A careful assessment of the client's cognitive status is essential because although she appears to be well oriented and capable of self-care, a more careful assessment may reveal that she has which of the following?
   1. A short-term memory loss
   2. A long-term memory loss
   3. Difficulty coping with stressors
   4. Lack of full range of motion

30. Which of the following best describes the term *smegma?*
   1. Loss of hair and baldness
   2. Cheesy-like substance secreted by the sebaceous glands
   3. Oily substance secreted by the sebaceous glands
   4. The reaction of bacteria with perspiration

31. Your client is a 58-year-old poorly nourished woman who was diagnosed with Alzheimer's disease 3 years ago. She has shown rapid deterioration and now is unable to care for any of her basic hygiene. Which nursing diagnosis is most appropriate?
   1. *Disturbed thought processes*
   2. *Disturbed sensory perception*
   3. *Activity intolerance*
   4. *Impaired physical mobility*

32. Your client is a 43-year-old female who has had severe rheumatoid arthritis for 15 years. She has severe limitations of both her lower and upper extremities. She has difficulty grasping objects because of malformation of her hand and fingers. Which nursing diagnosis is most appropriate?
   1. *Disturbed thought processes*
   2. *Disturbed sensory perception*
   3. *Activity intolerance*
   4. *Impaired physical mobility*

Copyright © 2004, Elsevier Science (USA). All Rights Reserved.

Restoring Physical Mobility

PURPOSE

This chapter introduces key concepts that relate to the nursing diagnoses *Impaired physical mobility* and *Activity intolerance*. It describes the concepts of the structure and function of the musculoskeletal system pertaining to mobility and discusses factors affecting mobility.

MATCHING

1. ____ flaccid

2. ____ hemiparesis

3. ____ hemiplegia

4. ____ isometric exercise

5. ____ isotonic exercise

6. ____ kyphosis

7. ____ paraparesis

8. ____ paraplegia

9. ____ PQRST model

10. ____ proprioception

11. ____ quadriparesis

12. ____ quadriplegia

13. ____ range-of-motion (ROM) exercises

14. ____ spastic

15. ____ synovium

a. the inner layer of the articular capsule surrounding a freely movable joint

b. sensation pertaining to stimuli originating from within the body regarding spatial position and muscular activity or to the sensory receptors that they activate

c. stands for: Provoking incidence, Quality, Region, Radiate, Relieve, Severity, and Timing of pain

d. an abnormal condition characterized by paralysis of the arms, legs, and trunk below the level of an associated injury to the spinal cord

e. a numbness or other abnormal or impaired sensation in all four limbs and the trunk

f. paralysis characterized by motor or sensory loss in the legs and trunk

g. paralysis of one side of the body

h. a numbness or other abnormal or impaired sensation experienced on only one side of the body that limits mobility and activities of daily living (ADLs)

i. an abnormal condition of the vertebral column characterized by increased convexity in the thoracic spine when viewed from the side

j. the state of being weak, soft, and flabby, lacking normal muscle tone, or having no ability to contract

k. contraction of skeletal muscles below the injury by reflex activity rather than by central nervous system control

l. a form of active exercise that increases muscle tension by applying pressure against stable resistance

m. form of active exercise in which the muscle contracts and moves

n. any body action (active or passive) involving the muscles, joints, and natural directional movements, such as abduction, extension, flexion, pronation, and rotation

o. a numbness or other abnormal or impaired sensation in the legs and trunk

TRUE OR FALSE

16. ____ Widening your base of support by moving your feet apart helps you to maintain stability.

17. ____ Postmenopausal women's vertebral bone mass increases and the thoracic spine becomes more convex, or curved.

Copyright © 2004, Elsevier Science (USA). All Rights Reserved.

18. _____ The most common congenital spinal deformity is scoliosis.

19. _____ Some medications have side effects that cause muscle atrophy.

20. _____ If a client can perform ADLs, a slight limitation of ROM is still unacceptable, especially for older adults.

21. _____ The client with *Impaired physical mobility* is at risk for injury from falls and fractures as a result of osteoporosis.

22. _____ For the postoperative client with a total knee replacement, a realistic intermediate outcome is that the client is expected to walk in the hospital room using a walker.

FILL-IN-THE-BLANKS

23. At about the age of 35 years _____ activity becomes greater than osteoblastic activity, which results in decreased bone that predisposes middle-aged and older adults to bone injury.

24. Muscle _____ causes weakness that can limit physical mobility.

25. An abnormal fixed position of the feet is _____ _____, or pigeon toe, a deformity that can worsen and delay physical development if not corrected.

26. The most common complaints associated with musculoskeletal health problems are pain, _____ _____, and inflammation.

27. _____ is a continuous grating sound caused by deterioration of a joint.

28. _____ and occupational therapists perform detailed assessments of muscle strength using various scales.

29. _____ nurses are specialists in helping clients return to or attain maximum function and a sense of well-being and independence.

EXERCISING YOUR CLINICAL JUDGMENT

30. Kristina Lasauskas, the client from this chapter's case study, had an open reduction and internal fixation to repair her fractured left hip. What nursing diagnosis would be most appropriate?
    1. *Impaired physical mobility*
    2. *Pain*
    3. *Activity intolerance*
    4. *Risk for injury*

31. Ms. Lasauskas needs help to learn how to increase her mobility skills after her surgery for a fractured left hip. Which one of the following discipline's primary role is improving clients' mobility skills?
    1. Rehabilitation nurse
    2. Physical therapist
    3. Occupational therapist
    4. Rehabilitation physician

32. Ms. Lasauskas will need ROM exercises while she is bedridden. What type of exercises are these?
    1. Isotonic
    2. Isokinetic
    3. Isometric
    4. Muscle toning

TEST YOURSELF

33. Pulling is usually easier than pushing, so pull clients toward you rather then push them. This can help do which one of the following?
    1. Reduce workload
    2. Decrease opposition from gravity
    3. Maintain stability
    4. Prevent muscle strain

34. Your client is having problems with her ankle. To assess her ankle's range of motion, which ROM exercises will you have her do?
    1. Flexion, extension, hyperextension
    2. Flexion, extension, abduction, adduction
    3. Plantar flexion, dorsiflexion, eversion, inversion
    4. External rotation, internal rotation

35. Your elderly client fell and fractured her hip and has degenerative arthritis in both knees. What nursing diagnosis would be most appropriate?
    1. *Impaired physical mobility*
    2. *Pain*
    3. *Activity intolerance*
    4. *Risk for injury*

36. Your teenage client has rheumatoid arthritis. She uses a walker to ambulate short distances, but relies on a wheelchair most of the time. She becomes very fatigued when walking. What nursing diagnosis would be most appropriate?
    1. *Impaired physical mobility*
    2. *Pain*
    3. *Activity intolerance*
    4. *Risk for injury*

37. Which one of the following discipline's primary role is improving clients' ADL abilities?
    1. Rehabilitation nurse
    2. Physical therapist
    3. Occupational therapist
    4. Rehabilitation physician

Copyright © 2004, Elsevier Science (USA). All Rights Reserved.

Preventing Disuse Syndrome

PURPOSE

This chapter discusses key concepts that relate to the nursing diagnosis *Risk for disuse syndrome*. It describes the physiological concepts underlying the diagnosis and the factors that may lead to immobility and disuse.

MATCHING

1. ____ atrophy

2. ____ bedrest

3. ____ contracture

4. ____ deep vein thrombosis

5. ____ disuse

6. ____ excoriation

7. ____ footdrop

8. ____ friction injury

9. ____ hypostatic pneumonia

10. ____ immobility

11. ____ interface pressure

12. ____ maceration

13. ____ orthostatic intolerance

14. ____ osteoporosis

15. ____ pressure ulcer

16. ____ pulmonary embolus

17. ____ renal calculi

18. ____ shear

19. ____ wrist drop

a. the inability to move the whole body or a body part

b. a prescribed or self-imposed restriction to bed for therapeutic reasons

c. a decrease in the size of a normally developed tissue or organ as a result of inactivity or diminished function

d. the abnormal shortening of muscle fibers or their associated connective tissue, resulting in resistance to stretching and eventually to flexion and, thereby resulting in permanent fixation

e. a contracture deformity in which the muscles of the anterior foot lengthen

f. a condition in which there is a decreased mass per unit volume of normally mineralized bone, primarily from a loss of calcium, that makes bones brittle and porous

g. a local defect or excavation of the surface of an organ or tissue that is produced by sloughing of necrotic inflammatory tissue created by impaired local circulation

h. pressure created in tissues that are compressed between the bones and a support surface by the weight of the body

i. a mechanical action in which an applied force exerted against the skin causes the tissue layers to slide in opposite but parallel directions, resulting in torn blood vessels

j. the epidermal layer of skin is rubbed off, possibly by a restraint, dressing, or tube

k. an injury to the epidermis caused by abrasion; scratching; a burn or chemicals, such as sweat; wound drainage; or feces or urine coming in contact with skin

l. a softening of the epidermis caused by prolonged contact with moisture, such as from a wet sheet or diaper

m. a drop in systolic blood pressure of 20 mm Hg or more and a drop in diastolic blood pressure of 10 mm Hg or more for 1 or 2 minutes after a client stands up

Copyright © 2004, Elsevier Science (USA). All Rights Reserved.

n. results when a piece of a deep vein thrombus breaks free, floats in the bloodstream to the pulmonary circulation, and lodges in a pulmonary blood vessel

o. the condition caused when a blood clot (thrombus) develops in the lumen of a deep leg vein, such as the tibial, popliteal, femoral, or iliac vein

p. an inflammation of the lungs, caused by stasis of secretions, that becomes a medium for bacterial growth

q. stones formed in the kidney when the excretion rate of calcium or other minerals is high, as when osteoclastic activity releases calcium from the bones during immobility

r. means to cease or decrease use of organs or body parts, to restrict activities, or to be immobile

s. a contracture of the wrist in the flexed position

TRUE OR FALSE

20. ____ Inactivity and immobility have a cyclic relationship with the development of complications.

21. ____ When muscles atrophy, they lose size and strength.

22. ____ Duration of immobilization of a client is not directly related to a higher risk of complications for the client of disuse.

23. ____ A pressure ulcer is a local defect or excavation of the surface of an organ or tissue that is produced by sloughing of necrotic inflammatory tissue creating impaired systemic circulation.

24. ____ Orthostatic intolerance is a rise in systolic blood pressure of 20 mm Hg or more and a drop in diastolic blood pressure of 10 mm Hg or more for 1 or 2 minutes after a client stands up.

25. ____ Clients who are at minimal *Risk for disuse* syndrome should be assessed every 4 to 6 hours.

26. ____ Constant contact with a bed made wet by perspiration causes maceration of the skin.

FILL-IN-THE-BLANKS

27. _____can affect a single body part or multiple interrelated body systems.

28. The _____ a person is immobile, the higher the risk of complication of disuse.

29. When a client is immobile, the body breaks down muscle mass to obtain _____.

30. Pressure _____ account for a large proportion of skin injuries that result from bed rest.

31. Low blood pressure and _____ _____ increase a client's risk of falling.

32. Stasis of the urine and infection increase the risk for _____ to form in the kidneys, renal pelvis, or urinary bladder.

33. You should assess and intervene every _____-_____ _____ with clients who have high *Risk for disuse syndrome.*

EXERCISING YOUR CLINICAL JUDGMENT

34. Mr. Jackson, the 48-year-old African-American with a compound fracture of the left tibia and a fractured left clavicle from this chapter's case study, develops a friction injury. This type of injury results from which of the following factors?
   1. The epidermal layer of skin is rubbed off.
   2. The client is neither very young nor very old.
   3. There is a decrease in range of motion.
   4. There is maximal inactivity of long duration.

35. Mr. Jackson has moderate inactivity of moderate duration, is middle-aged, has normal to slight increased body weight, no chronic illnesses, minimal discomfort, and low environmental risk. Your client is at moderate *Risk for disuse* syndrome. How often should you assess and intervene with this client?
   1. Every 4 to 6 hours
   2. Every 2 to 4 hours
   3. Every 1 to 2 hours
   4. Every shift

36. You encourage Mr. Jackson to exercise his right arm and leg against resistance three times daily. Which nursing diagnosis does Mr. Jackson have?
   1. *Ineffective role performance*
   2. *Disturbed sensory perception*
   3. *Risk for disuse syndrome*
   4. *Self-care deficit*

TEST YOURSELF

37. Your client has been immobile for several weeks. Once he begins ambulating he is more susceptible to ambulation problems and injury caused by what?
   1. Footdrop
   2. Contracture
   3. Osteoporosis
   4. Falling

Copyright © 2004, Elsevier Science (USA). All Rights Reserved.

38. Your client has a deformity that involves flexion of the wrist and fingers and opposition of the thumb. You would state in intershift report that the client has which of the following?
    1. Hand drop
    2. Wrist drop
    3. Osteoporosis
    4. Ankylosis

39. Your client has softening of the epidermis caused by prolonged contact with a wet sheet. What type of injury is this?
    1. Maceration
    2. Shear
    3. Friction injury
    4. Excoriation

40. There are two purposes that are unique to assessing the immobile client. One is to detect the risk of complication of immobility. The second purpose is to determine which of the following?
    1. The client's needs
    2. How much assistance the client will need to manage the activities of daily living and prevent complications
    3. The client's emotional well-being
    4. The client's level of understanding of his or her situation

41. To relieve pressure, how often do you turn the client to a new position?
    1. Every 1 to 2 hours
    2. Every hour
    3. Twice a shift
    4. Every 3 hours

Copyright © 2004, Elsevier Science (USA). All Rights Reserved.

Supporting Respiratory Function

33

PURPOSE

The purpose of this chapter is to review anatomy and physiology of the respiratory system and to introduce you to basic respiratory nursing measures. You will learn to recognize the signs and symptoms of respiratory distress and intervene to improve respiratory function. Additionally you will be introduced to some advance procedures, such as managing a chest tube, suctioning the airway, and caring for a tracheostomy.

MATCHING

1. ____ bronchospasm

2. ____ chest percussion

3. ____ chest physiotherapy

4. ____ cough

5. ____ cyanosis

6. ____ diaphragmatic (abdominal) breathing

7. ____ dyspnea

8. ____ endotracheal tube

9. ____ hemoptysis

10. ____ hypercapnia

11. ____ hyperventilation

12. ____ hypoventilation

13. ____ hypoxemia

14. ____ hypoxia

15. ____ incentive spirometer

16. ____ postural drainage

17. ____ pulse oximeter

18. ____ pursed-lip breathing

19. ____ respiration

20. ____ sputum

21. ____ ventilation

22. ____ vibration

a. a bluish color to the skin that results from the concentration of deoxygenated hemoglobin close to the surface of the skin

b. spasm of the smooth muscles of the bronchi and/or the bronchioles that results in decreased airway diameter

c. using cupped hands to rhythmically clap on the chest wall over various segments of the lungs to mobilize secretions

d. a sudden audible, forceful expulsion of air from the lungs, usually an involuntary, reflexive action in response to an irritant

e. coughing and spitting up blood as a result of bleeding from any part of the lower respiratory tract

f. a catheter passed through the nose or mouth into the trachea for the purpose of establishing an airway

g. high carbon dioxide level in the blood, usually resulting from failure of the lungs to remove carbon dioxide

h. breathing in which the majority of ventilatory work is accomplished by the diaphragm and abdominal muscles; deliberate use of the diaphragm and abdominal muscles to control breathing

i. an approach to mobilizing and draining secretions from gravity-dependent areas of the lung that uses a combination of postural drainage, chest percussion, and vibration

j. the subjective sensation of difficulty in breathing

k. increase in the rate and depth of breathing, clinically defined as $PaCO_2$ less than 35 mm Hg

Copyright © 2004, Elsevier Science (USA). All Rights Reserved.

l. a method of measuring the oxygen saturation of functional hemoglobin in the blood

m. a technique in which the client assumes one or more positions that will facilitate the drainage of secretions from the bronchial airways

n. a technique of mouth breathing that creates slight resistance to exhalation by contracting the lips to reduce the size of the opening, thus maintaining an even reduction of intrathoracic pressure during exhalation

o. deficient oxygenation of the blood

p. mucus secreted from the lungs, bronchi, and trachea; may include epithelial cells, bacteria, and debris

q. a device that provides a visual goal for and measurement of inspiration, thus encouraging the client to execute and sustain maximal inspiration

r. decrease in the rate and depth of breathing, clinically defined as $PaCO_2$ greater than 45 mm Hg

s. the process of exchanging air between the ambient air and the lungs; *pulmonary ventilation* refers to the total exchange of air, whereas *alveolar ventilation* refers to the effective ventilation of the alveoli

t. a technique of chest physiotherapy whereby the chest wall is set in motion by oscillating movements of the hands or a vibrator for the purpose of mobilizing secretions

u. the exchange of oxygen and carbon dioxide between the atmosphere and the cells of the body; a series of metabolic activities by which living cells break down carbohydrates, amino acids, and fats to produce energy in the form of ATP (adenosine triphosphate)

v. deficient oxygenation of body tissues

TRUE OR FALSE

23. ____ The accessory muscles of respiration become more active during forceful expiration.

24. ____ The work of breathing is directly related to the amount of airway resistance.

25. ____ Tidal volume is the amount of air inhaled with a deep inspiration.

26. ____ Oxygen and carbon dioxide are exchanged through the alveolar membrane by the passive process of diffusion.

27. ____ Fowler's position is the position of optimum ventilation/perfusion ratio.

28. ____ In the older adult, decreased compliance and elasticity increase the risk for respiratory complications during illness or surgery.

29. ____ Nicotine patches have a 50% success rate in helping people quit smoking.

30. ____ Fractured ribs are a type of obstructive respiratory disease.

31. ____ Asthma is more common where there is a history of asthma in the family.

32. ____ Ambulation is an efficient, noninvasive, inexpensive method of stimulating respiration.

33. ____ Endotracheal suctioning is a sterile procedure without regard to the client's condition or setting.

34. ____ Oxygen therapy is given in the lowest possible dose to maintain arterial oxygen saturation above 90%.

FILL-IN-THE-BLANK

35. The primary muscle of respiration is the _____.

36. _____ _____ is the tendency of the lungs to return to a nonstretched state.

37. _____ is a lipoprotein secreted by the alveolar epithelium and acts like a detergent to reduce the surface tension and hold the alveoli open.

38. _____ stimulates the production of surfactant.

39. _____ _____ is any surface of the airways that contains air but does not participate in gas exchange.

40. The _____ is the opening at the top of the larynx between the resting vocal cords.

41. A _____ _____ _____ is the diagnostic test that provides information about the oxygen-carrying capacity of the blood.

42. The _____ _____ _____ is the volume of air forcefully (with maximum effort) exhaled after a maximum inhalation.

43. The pulse oximetry measurement is used to ensure that oxygen saturation is maintained above _____ %.

44. _____ describes the client rendered insensitive to painful stimuli by reducing the level of consciousness with a narcotic or anesthetic. This client has rapid shallow breathing.

45. _____, _____ sputum is difficult to cough out and may be associated with dehydration.

Copyright © 2004, Elsevier Science (USA). All Rights Reserved.

46. The client with pain from a high abdominal surgical incision is at risk for the nursing diagnosis of _____ _____ _____.

47. Cyanosis represents the presence of increased amounts of _____ _____ in the blood.

48. _____ is a medication used to reverse the action of narcotics, thus stimulating respiration.

EXERCISING YOUR CLINICAL JUDGMENT

Mrs. Wilheim, the client introduced in the chapter's case study, has been admitted to the hospital with a diagnosis of pneumonia. Her physician orders include antibiotic therapy and oxygen therapy.

49. Mrs. Wilheim is placed on oxygen via nasal cannula, a low-flow oxygen delivery system. Which of the following statements best describes this therapy?
    1. The wall-mounted oxygen flow meter delivers 35% to 45% oxygen to the nasal cannula.
    2. The client supplements the flow of oxygen with room air to maintain the minute ventilation.
    3. A low-flow system can only deliver 28% oxygen.
    4. 100% oxygen from the wall is mixed precisely with room air to deliver the ordered percentage of oxygen.

50. Mrs. Wilheim is hypoventilating because of her disease process. Which of the following pieces of client data best fits the definition of hypoventilation?
    1. Respiratory rate of 36, with visible chest wall movement in the upper third of the chest
    2. A measured tidal volume of 500 with a rate of 12
    3. Arterial carbon dioxide level of 43, oxygen saturation of 94%
    4. Respiratory rate of 10, no dyspnea, color good, skin warm and dry

51. Mrs. Wilheim is subsequently given medication via metered-dose inhaler to enhance her breathing. The nurse teaching her to correctly use a metered-dose inhaler would instruct her to do which of the following?
    1. Activate the inhaler and then take a deep breath
    2. Take a deep breath and then activate the inhaler
    3. Simultaneously activate the inhaler and take a deep breath
    4. Activate the inhaler, close the mouth, and take a deep breath

TEST YOURSELF

52. Your client had a thoracentesis 30 minutes ago. He is complaining of shortness of breath. You listen to his lungs. Which finding indicates the possibility of the complication of atelectasis?
    1. Bilateral crackles (rales) in the bases
    2. Diminished breath sounds on the side where the thoracentesis was performed
    3. Harsh sonorous sounds over the bifurcation of the bronchi
    4. Wet, bubbling sounds over the midsternum

53. Your client is having an asthma attack. You hear wheezes throughout the lung fields. You can attribute the sounds to which of the following?
    1. Mucus in the bronchioles
    2. Atelectasis
    3. Bronchospasms
    4. Inflammation of the pleura

54. A client who has a dry, hacking cough and wheezes throughout the lung fields would be given which of the following nursing diagnoses?
    1. *Ineffective airway clearance*
    2. *Ineffective breathing pattern*
    3. *Impaired gas exchange*
    4. *Obstructive airway disease*

55. Your postoperative client has an order for an incentive spirometer treatment q2h for the 72 hours following surgery. He asks you why he needs this treatment when his surgery was on his abdomen. Which of the following responses is best?
    1. "It will help you use all of your lungs when you breathe and prevent a respiratory infection."
    2. "It helps you maintain a maximal inspiration, thus preventing atelectasis."
    3. "It will increase the perfusion to your lungs for better arterial oxygen saturation."
    4. "It will increase the blood flow to your lungs so you can get more oxygen from the air that you breathe."

56. Your client with chronic obstructive pulmonary disease has chronic inflammation in her lungs. She is taking a corticosteroid by metered-dose inhaler. She asks why she can't just take a pill. Which of the following would be the most accurate response?
    1. "Your doctor prefers a metered-dose inhaler."
    2. "You can use the metered-dose inhaler anytime you need it."
    3. "The medication in a pill form won't reach your lungs."
    4. "You are less likely to have the complication of failure of your adrenal glands to produce corticosteroids."

Copyright © 2004, Elsevier Science (USA). All Rights Reserved.

57. You observe all of the following in your client with a chest tube. Select the finding that represents the most serious complication of a chest tube.
    1. 100 ml of serosanguineous drainage in an 8-hour period
    2. Itching under the pressure dressing around the chest tube
    3. Air from the pleural space bubbling in the water-sealed drainage system
    4. Sucking air into the pleural space through the chest tube

58. Which of the following would be the primary purpose of pursed-lip breathing?
    1. Increase the resistance to expiration to maintain functional residual volume
    2. Help the client focus on the respiration during times of stress
    3. Increase the inspiratory capacity thus improving exercise tolerance
    4. Produce the relaxation response during times of dyspnea

59. Which of the following would be the primary reason for a client to learn diaphragmatic breathing?
    1. Increase the strength and use of the diaphragm for exhalation
    2. Increase the strength and use of the diaphragm for inhalation
    3. Produce the relaxation response and reduce stress
    4. Reduce the strength and use of the accessory muscles of respiration

60. You are suctioning the client's airway through a tracheostomy. Which of the following actions represents a correct nursing action during this procedure?
    1. Apply suction continuously as you enter the airway.
    2. Apply suction intermittently as you enter the airway.
    3. Apply suction continuously as you exit the airway.
    4. Apply suction intermittently as you exit the airway.

61. For which of the following reasons is the Yankauer tip suction device used for safety in oral suctioning?
    1. The tip has multiple openings thus preventing damage to the oral mucosa.
    2. It can be attached only to low-suction devices.
    3. The hard plastic catheter cannot be swallowed by the client.
    4. The openings are not large enough to cause mucosal damage.

62. Which of the following represents the primary principle in assisting the client to clear the airway?
    1. To use the most aggressive procedure first to reduce the time needed for treatment
    2. To use the least invasive procedure necessary to produce the desired results
    3. To avoid invasive suctioning until the secretions are life threatening
    4. To suction when the level of need is preventive

63. The most serious complication of suction is represented by which of the following data?
    1. Streaks of blood in the sputum
    2. Oxygen saturation of 88%
    3. Large amount of watery sputum
    4. Moderate amounts of yellow sputum

Copyright © 2004, Elsevier Science (USA). All Rights Reserved.

34

Supporting Cardiovascular Function

PURPOSE

This chapter discusses concepts of and factors affecting cardiovascular function. It uses the nursing process as a framework to discuss management of *decreased tissue perfusion* as a result of common cardiovascular problems.

MATCHING

1. ____ afterload
2. ____ antidiuretic hormone
3. ____ atherosclerosis
4. ____ baroreceptors
5. ____ bradycardia
6. ____ cardiac output
7. ____ claudication
8. ____ diastole
9. ____ dysrhythmia
10. ____ edema
11. ____ inotropic agent
12. ____ ischemia
13. ____ necrosis
14. ____ preload
15. ____ stroke volume
16. ____ systole
17. ____ tachycardia
18. ____ viscosity

a. specialized cells located in the aorta and carotid bodies that detect pressure changes in the vascular system

b. cramplike pains in the calves caused by poor circulation of blood to the leg muscles

c. a heart rate above 100 beats per minute

d. a decreased supply of oxygenated blood to tissues

e. contraction of the ventricles

f. the pressure against which the left ventricle pumps

g. a hormonal compensatory mechanism that is also called vasopressin

h. the amount of blood in the left ventricle immediately before contraction

i. the amount of blood pumped by the ventricles in 1 minute

j. refers to the relaxation of the ventricles

k. the relative ability of a fluid to flow that results from the thickness of the fluid

l. abnormalities of heart rate or rhythm

m. an abnormal accumulation of fluid in the interstitial spaces of tissues, commonly known as swelling

n. localized death of tissues caused by disease, oxygen deficit, or injury

o. medication that increases the contractility of the heart muscle, thereby increasing cardiac output

p. a pathological condition in which fat and plaque form deposits on the intimal (inner) surface of the arteries

q. the amount of blood ejected from the heart with each contraction

r. a heart rate less than 60 beats per minute

TRUE OR FALSE

19. ____ Highly viscous blood encounters more resistance while moving through blood vessels.

Copyright © 2004, Elsevier Science (USA). All Rights Reserved.

20. ____ Starling's law indicates that stronger recoil of cardiac muscle tissue produces weaker stroke volume.

21. ____ Elevated blood glucose is a modifiable risk factor for cardiovascular disease.

22. ____ Nicotine produces vasodilatation, which increases blood flow to tissues, and increases the oxygen-carrying capacity of hemoglobin.

23. ____ Women have an increased incidence of Raynaud's disease, whereas men are more likely to have Buerger's disease.

24. ____ Atherosclerotic plaque deposits create a rough spot on the normally smooth inner surface of the blood vessel.

25. ____ Bacterial and viral infections of the heart are minor problems that leave no permanent heart damage as a result.

26. ____ Stress increases the heart rate and blood pressure, which, in turn, raise the body's oxygen demands.

27. ____ Excessive intake of high-fat foods can lead to elevated serum cholesterol levels.

28. ____ Lack of circulation destroys nerves and impairs motor function in the involved extremity.

FILL-IN-THE-BLANKS

29. The average cardiac output is _____ to _____ liters per minute.

30. _____ and _____ are stimulants that increase heart rate and oxygen demand.

31. The primary effect of aging as a developmental factor on the circulation is the development of _____.

32. Hypertension is a condition in which the blood pressure is persistently higher than _____ /_____ mm Hg.

33. A _____ _____ is the blockage of a blood vessel in the brain through thrombus, embolus, or hemorrhage, which results in ischemia or death of brain tissue distal to the insult.

34. Fluid in the lungs is a prominent symptom in _____ -sided heart failure.

35. _____ is needed to manufacture oxygen-carrying hemoglobin molecules.

36. Clients who take _____ and warfarin have a dangerous risk of bleeding.

37. Antihistamines and appetite suppressants are contraindicated for clients with hypertension because they cause _____.

38. Lifestyle choices such as _____, _____, and _____ have direct effects on circulation.

EXERCISING YOUR CLINICAL JUDGMENT

Mr. Yoder, the man introduced in the chapter's case study, is a 74-year-old Amish client who has a medical diagnosis of angina pectoris and a nursing diagnosis of *Ineffective cardiopulmonary tissue perfusion*. He was admitted 2 days ago with chest pain and underwent cardiac catheterization yesterday. You are assigned to take care of Mr. Yoder today and must develop and implement a teaching plan before his discharge, which is planned for later this afternoon.

39. To help Mr. Yoder conserve energy in order to decrease oxygen demand, you should encourage him to do which of the following?
    1. Take rest breaks between daily activities such as eating, bathing, and walking.
    2. Do all of his chores early in the morning provided he has had a good night's sleep.
    3. Save chores for late in the day so endurance will be greater.
    4. Stop all exertional activities and turn over responsibility for them to his son.

40. You would encourage Mr. Yoder to limit which of the following food items that typically has a high salt content?
    1. Vegetables
    2. Freshwater fish
    3. Sauces
    4. Fruits

41. Knowing that Mr. Yoder is being discharged with a prescription for an antihypertensive medication, which of the following general teaching points would you include in a discussion with him?
    1. Take the medication when eating a heavy meal.
    2. Wear slippers or shoes at all times.
    3. The medication should be taken whenever chest pain occurs.
    4. Rise out of bed or out of a chair slowly.

42. In teaching Mr. Yoder to avoid the Valsalva maneuver, you would tell him it is important to avoid which of the following activities?
    1. Drinking lots of fluids
    2. Bearing down hard when having a bowel movement
    3. Walking up and down stairs
    4. Lying flat in bed

Copyright © 2004, Elsevier Science (USA). All Rights Reserved.

TEST YOURSELF

43. To determine the presence of jugular vein distention, the nurse would take which of the following actions?
    1. Raise the head of the bed to 45 degrees
    2. Turn the client onto the right side
    3. Lay the client supine in bed
    4. Turn the client onto the left side

44. A client has had a cardiac catheterization using the right femoral artery as the access site. The nurse would report which of the following peripheral vascular findings in the client's right leg following the procedure?
    1. Strong palpable pedal pulse
    2. Pink skin
    3. Warmth
    4. Numbness and tingling

45. The nurse would assess for which of the following peripheral vascular manifestations in a client with venous disease of the lower extremities?
    1. Pale, cool skin
    2. Decreased pulses
    3. Edema
    4. Tingling and burning sensations

46. A nurse has signed out a unit of blood from the blood bank at 2:00 PM. The unit must be hung by which of the following times in order to prevent bacterial contamination of the unit?
    1. 6:00 PM
    2. 4:00 PM
    3. 3:30 PM
    4. 2:20 PM

47. A nurse who has administered care to a client in shock interprets that the shock state is resolving. The nurse bases this conclusion on which of the following pieces of client data?
    1. Urine output 45 ml/hour
    2. Pulse rate 128 beats per minute
    3. Blood pressure 92/48 mm Hg
    4. Neurological confusion

Copyright © 2004, Elsevier Science (USA). All Rights Reserved.

Managing Sleep and Rest

PURPOSE

This chapter introduces you to concepts central to normal sleep and rest, and the variations from normal that can occur. It describes how to use the nursing process to assist the client in meeting personal needs for sleep and rest.

MATCHING

1. ____ bruxism
2. ____ circadian rhythm
3. ____ dyssomnia
4. ____ hypersomnia
5. ____ hypnotic
6. ____ insomnia
7. ____ multiple sleep latency test
8. ____ narcolepsy
9. ____ nightmare
10. ____ nonrapid eye movement (NREM) sleep
11. ____ obstructive sleep apnea
12. ____ parasomnia
13. ____ polysomnography
14. ____ rapid eye movement (REM) sleep
15. ____ rest
16. ____ restless legs syndrome
17. ____ sedative
18. ____ sleep
19. ____ sleep deprivation
20. ____ sleep enuresis
21. ____ sleep terrors
22. ____ slow-wave sleep
23. ____ somnambulism
24. ____ sundowning
25. ____ zeitgeber

a. a biorhythmic pattern that is regularly repeated at 24-hour intervals

b. the state that results from a person not getting enough sleep

c. difficulty initiating or maintaining sleep

d. occur during slow-wave sleep and are characterized by arousal, agitation, and signs of sympathetic nervous system activity, such as dilated pupils, sweating, tachypnea, and tachycardia

e. a sleep disorder manifested by periodic cessation of airflow at the nose and mouth during inspiration, which arouses the person from sleep

f. the continuous measurement and recording of physiological activity during sleep by using electroencephalogram, electrooculogram, electrocardiogram, and electromyogram.

g. a reversible behavioral state in which consciousness, activity of the skeletal muscles, and metabolism are depressed

h. a direct, objective measure of sleepiness used to evaluate excessive somnolence and daytime sleepiness.

i. a state of being physically and mentally relaxed while being awake and alert

j. is characterized by high-voltage EEG activity and a high arousal threshold, which can make it difficult to arouse the sleeper

k. a parasomnia characterized by violent, repetitive grinding of the teeth that occurs during the lighter stages of sleep or during partial arousals.

l. a slow-wave sleep parasomnia associated with stereotypical "sleepwalking" behaviors

m. any sleep disturbance that involves the amount, quality, or timing of sleep

Copyright © 2004, Elsevier Science (USA). All Rights Reserved.

n. a parasomnia characterized by bed-wetting during sleep

o. a sleep disruption involving the nocturnal exacerbation of disruptive behaviors and agitation associated with clients who have dementia

p. a state in which a quiet brain functions in an active body

q. a striking hypersomnia characterized by abnormal sleep tendencies as well as by pathological REM sleep, manifested as excessive daytime sleepiness, disturbed nighttime sleep, cataplexy, sleep paralysis, and hypnagogic hallucinations

r. sleep disorders that are not difficulties with sleep themselves, but rather abnormal movements and behaviors that occur during sleep

s. a drug that acts on the CNS to shorten sleep onset, reduce nighttime wakefulness, or decrease anxiety when insomnia is associated with increased anxiety

t. a vivid or frightening dream that occurs during REM sleep, awakens the sleeper, and can be vividly recalled

u. is a drug that exerts a soothing, tranquilizing effect on the CNS, resulting in a shortened sleep onset and the alleviation of anxiety

v. is a sleep disorder characterized by excessive sleepiness

w. an intrinsic sleep disorder characterized by intense, abnormal, lower extremity sensations and irresistible leg movements that delay sleep onset

x. a state in which a highly active brain functions in an immobilized body

y. adjust the human body's internal clock to a 24-hour solar day

TRUE OR FALSE

26. ____ Wrist actigraphs are a newer means of measuring sleep in the client's home by application of a bracelet that records wrist movements that signal restlessness during sleep.

27. ____ A client who is physically rested is therefore also mentally rested.

28. ____ An electroencephalogram (EEG) can be used to distinguish among coma, sleep, and wakefulness when other assessment results are inconclusive.

29. ____ Current thought is that a complex network of neurons passing through the medulla, pons, midbrain, thalamus, hypothalamus, and basal forebrain maintains homeostatic balance between sleep and wakefulness.

30. ____ Restless legs syndrome is an extrinsic sleep disorder.

31. ____ A person experiencing a night terror should be awakened by others nearby.

32. ____ The half-life of nicotine is 1 to 2 hours.

33. ____ Chronic fatigue syndrome is a long-standing fatigue that lasts for 6 months or more.

FILL-IN-THE-BLANKS

34. A _____ is an environmental trigger or synchronizer that adjusts the body's internal clock to a 24-hour day.

35. _____ is the "hormone of darkness" that regulates the circadian phase of sleep.

36. A person should avoid excess coffee, tea, or chocolate near bedtime because they contain the stimulant _____.

37. ICU psychosis is an iatrogenic complication that is strongly correlated with _____ sleep deprivation in ICUs.

38. The sleep-wake cycle is fully developed by the age of _____.

39. _____ is one of the few sleep disorders with a demonstrated genetic link.

40. A person with sleep apnea should avoid sleeping on the _____.

41. The only spice or herb that has been shown in some studies to improve the subjective quality of sleep is _____.

EXERCISING YOUR CLINICAL JUDGMENT

Ms. Weiss, the woman introduced in the chapter's case study, is experiencing transient situational insomnia that she attributes to a new job and enrollment in graduate school courses. Personal habits include drinking a glass of wine to help with sleep, and smoking cigarettes and drinking coffee throughout the day. The nurse practitioner has asked you to counsel Ms. Weiss about nonprescription treatments for her sleep disorder.

Copyright © 2004, Elsevier Science (USA). All Rights Reserved.

42. Knowing that caffeine has stimulant properties, you would encourage Ms. Weiss to refrain from drinking coffee after which of the following times?
    1. Noon
    2. 2 PM
    3. 4 PM
    4. 8 PM

43. To reduce the interference of nicotine with Ms. Weiss's sleep, you would advise her to continue to try to have the last cigarette no later than:
    1. Midmorning.
    2. Lunchtime.
    3. Suppertime.
    4. An hour before bed.

44. When discussing the Bootzin technique with Ms. Weiss, you would include which of the following points?
    1. Adjust the alarm clock nightly to a time that allows for 8 hours of continuous sleep.
    2. If you cannot get to sleep after 30 minutes of trying, get up and go into another room until sleepy.
    3. Take a nap at midday to make up for sleep lost the previous night.
    4. Go to bed at the same time each night, regardless of whether you feel sleepy.

45. You are instructing Ms. Weiss about progressive relaxation techniques as a method to promote sleep onset. Which of the following points would you include?
    1. The exercises should be practiced for 45 to 60 minutes before going to bed.
    2. They should be used only at bedtime but not during the night if wakefulness occurs.
    3. They are not to be used in conjunction with deep breathing exercises.
    4. Relaxation begins with voluntary muscles in the feet and progresses upward to the face.

TEST YOURSELF

46. A client reports an inability to fall asleep, which is followed by awakening at night and a sense of not feeling well rested in the morning. The nurse interprets that these symptoms are defining characteristics of which of the following nursing diagnoses?
    1. *Fatigue*
    2. *Disturbed sleep pattern*
    3. *Anxiety*
    4. *Altered thought processes*

47. The nurse who is planning behavioral outcomes for a client who has a problem with interrupted sleep would include which of the following suggestions?
    1. Not eat heavy or fat-filled foods just before going to sleep
    2. Refrain from drinking milk before bedtime.
    3. Drink a glass of wine or beer just prior to bedtime.
    4. Keep a bedside lamp on during the night.

48. When teaching a client cognitive strategies to reduce insomnia, the nurse would encourage the client to spend 20 minutes reflecting on daytime activities and achievements:
    1. just after getting home from work, such as around 4 PM.
    2. just prior to going to bed.
    3. just after getting into bed for the night.
    4. in the early evening after dinner.

49. The nurse would encourage the client who has an order for a prn sleep medication to take it:
    1. just after supper.
    2. two hours before going to bed.
    3. shortly before going to bed.
    4. an hour after going to bed if not successful falling asleep.

50. The nurse would evaluate that interventions to treat a *Disturbed sleep pattern* were most effective if the client states:
    1. compliance with the interventions prescribed.
    2. feeling well rested after sleep.
    3. obtaining 4 hours of uninterrupted sleep per night.
    4. using at least half of the methods suggested by the nurse.

Copyright © 2004, Elsevier Science (USA). All Rights Reserved.

Managing Pain

PURPOSE

This chapter discusses key concepts that relate to the nursing diagnoses *Chronic pain* and *Pain*. It describes the physiological concepts supporting pain-related nursing diagnoses. It also describes pathophysiological, cognitive, affective, sensory, cultural, environmental, and other variables that affect the pain experience.

MATCHING

1. ____ acute pain

2. ____ adjuvant analgesic

3. ____ agonist analgesic

4. ____ analgesia

5. ____ antagonist

6. ____ atypical analgesic

7. ____ breakthrough pain

8. ____ chronic pain

9. ____ endorphin

10. ____ epidural analgesia

11. ____ equianalgesia

12. ____ first pass effect

13. ____ gate control theory

14. ____ intrathecal analgesia

15. ____ mixed agonist-antagonist analgesic

16. ____ modulation

17. ____ neuropathic pain

18. ____ nociception

19. ____ nociceptive pain

20. ____ nociceptor

21. ____ nonopioid analgesic

22. ____ opioid analgesic

23. ____ opioid naive

24. ____ opioid receptor

25. ____ pain

26. ____ pain behavior

27. ____ patient-controlled analgesia

28. ____ physical dependence

29. ____ psychological dependence

30. ____ referred pain

31. ____ rescue dose

32. ____ somatic pain

33. ____ suffering

34. ____ tolerance

35. ____ visceral pain

a. an unpleasant sensory and emotional experience associated with actual and potential tissue damage

b. the process of transmitting a pain signal from a site of tissue damage to areas of the brain where perception occurs

c. pain transmitted from a site of injury to the higher brain centers along an intact nervous system

d. the transmission of a pain signal from the site of injury to the higher brain centers via a nervous system that has been temporarily or permanently damaged in some way

e. well-located pain, usually bone or spinal metastases or from injury to cutaneous or deep tissues

f. poorly localized pain

g. pain experienced at a site distant from the injured tissue

h. an internal or external restraining of the nociceptive process that inhibits transmission of the pain signal at any place along the transmission pathway

Copyright © 2004, Elsevier Science (USA). All Rights Reserved.

i. a portion of a nerve cell to which an opioid or opiate-like substance can bind

j. morphine-like drug that attaches to an opioid receptor and produces analgesia by blocking substance P

k. a drug that provides analgesia at the peripheral level by a mechanism other than the opioid receptor sites

l. an opioid that stimulates activity at an opioid receptor to produce analgesia

m. blocks activity at *mu* and *kappa* opioid receptors by displacing opioid analgesics that are currently attached

n. formulation that attaches to both the *kappa* and *mu* receptor sites

o. an involuntary physiological phenomenon that occurs after repeated exposure to an opioid analgesic; it involves a decreased-level pain relief despite a stable or escalating opioid dosage

p. an involuntary physiological phenomenon that occurs after repeated exposure to an opioid analgesic

q. a chronic disorder demonstrated by overwhelming involvement with obtaining and using a drug for its mind-altering effects

r. anything a person says or does that infers the presence of pain

s. short-term, self-limiting pain with a probable duration of less than 6 months

t. long-term, constant or recurring pain without an anticipated or predictable end and a duration of more than 6 months

u. drugs not primarily indicated for pain but used to treat specific types of pain

v. a catheter is placed in the subarachnoid space between the dura mater and the spinal cord to allow immediate drug diffusion into the cerebrospinal fluid

w. a catheter is placed between the spinal vertebrae and the dura mater to allow the diffusion of an analgesic drug across the dura mater into the cerebrospinal fluid

x. a drug-delivery approach that uses an external infusion pump to deliver an opioid dose on a "client-demand" basis

y. intermittent episodes of pain that occur despite continued use of an analgesic

z. as-needed dose of an immediate-release analgesic in response to breakthrough pain and in addition to the scheduled analgesic dosage

aa. the dosage that provides the same amount of pain relief independent of the drug or the route

bb. the partial metabolism of opioid analgesics by the liver before they reach the systemic circulation, thereby resulting in a decrease in opioid availability (dosage)

cc. those who have had minimal or no exposure to opioid analgesics

dd. any medication that may increase analgesic efficacy, thus allowing for a smaller opioid dosage

ee. the primary afferent fibers that initiate the pain experience when stimulated by tissue damage

ff. a group of internally secreted opiate-like substances released by a signal from the cerebral cortex

gg. unpleasant emotional response to pain

hh. a reduction in the perception or experience of pain

ii. hypothesizes an alteration in the transmission of the ascending pain signal by a spinal gating mechanism located in the dorsal horn; the pain signal may be inhibited or facilitated by multiple variables

TRUE OR FALSE

36. ____ Pain is primarily a protective mechanism, but it is also a complex biopsychosocial phenomenon.

37. ____ Visceral pain is well-localized pain, usually from bone or spinal metastases or from injury to cutaneous or deep tissues.

38. ____ A single disorder may have components of both nociceptive and neuropathic pain.

39. ____ Educating a client about what to expect during a painful procedure decreases the pain's intensity and controls pain behaviors.

40. ____ Pain is the actual physical sensation of discomfort, whereas suffering is the unpleasant emotional response.

41. ____ Pain is a normal part of aging.

42. ____ The administration schedule of analgesia should be based on the known half-life of the drug.

FILL-IN-THE-BLANKS

43. Pain functions as a _____ tool, an assessment variable, and a measure of _____ interventions.

Copyright © 2004, Elsevier Science (USA). All Rights Reserved.

44. _____ pain is experienced at a site distant from the injured tissue.

45. Behavioral expressions of pain are _____ from others.

46. _____ pain can quickly deplete a person's physical and emotional resources, immobilize the person, and lead to physical disability and subsequent loss of employment.

47. Once you choose a _____ _____ _____ for a client, continue to use the same scale throughout your ongoing assessment to keep the responses as comparable as possible over time.

48. Clients with _____ pain commonly have trouble finding adequate words to describe the sensation.

49. Nonmalignant etiologies are more likely to produce _____ pain, which tends to be difficult to treat and, at times, more disabling than cancer pain.

EXERCISING YOUR CLINICAL JUDGMENT

50. Mr. Joseph Valdez, the client from the chapter's case study, was born in Mexico City. He has recurrent gastric carcinoma and he hurts most of the time. His brothers told him to be tough and that he could "beat this thing." They were encouraging him to remain stoic even in the presence of severe pain. This is an example of which of the following?
    1. Religious beliefs
    2. Psychosocial modifiers
    3. Cultural norms
    4. Aggravating and relieving variables

51. Mr. Valdez is being admitted to an oncology unit for epidural catheter placement. He is experiencing unrelieved and severe pain. Which of the following nursing diagnoses would be appropriate?
    1. *Ineffective individual coping*
    2. *Hopelessness*
    3. *Pain*
    4. *Chronic pain*

52. Mr. Valdez experiences breakthrough pain. Which of the following actions would you take to treat him with rescue dosing?
    1. Call his physician and request he receive a more effective analgesic
    2. Give him a one-time extra dose of his analgesic
    3. Change the schedule of his analgesic to be more effective
    4. Give him as-needed doses of an immediate-release analgesic in addition to the scheduled analgesic dosage

TEST YOURSELF

53. Which type of pain is described as squeezing, pressure, cramping, distention, or deep stretching?
    1. Somatic
    2. Visceral
    3. Referred
    4. Neuropathic

54. Your client develops withdrawal symptoms if the opioid is abruptly withdrawn or an opioid antagonist is administered. This is considered which of the following?
    1. Tolerance
    2. Physical dependence
    3. Psychological dependence
    4. Pseudo-addiction

55. You use a pain rating scale that is a 10 cm horizontal line. At its left endpoint is written *No pain at all*. At its right endpoint is written *Worst pain imaginable*. What type of pain rating scale is this?
    1. Self-report rating scale
    2. Verbal descriptor scale
    3. Numerical rating scale
    4. A visual analog scale

56. In the frail elderly the most sensitive indicator of pain may be which of the following?
    1. Crying out in pain
    2. Moaning
    3. An observed decrease in the client's usual level of functioning
    4. Facial grimacing

57. If your client is receiving an opioid analgesic for acute or chronic pain and her respiratory rate is significantly affected (fewer than 8 breaths per minute), the appropriate intervention is which of the following?
    1. Stop the opioid analgesic until the respiratory rate returns to normal.
    2. Slowly push intravenously 0.4 mg of naloxone (Narcan) that has been diluted in normal saline to equal 10 ml until an adequate respiratory rate returns but pain relief remains intact.
    3. Quickly push intravenously 0.4 mg of naloxone (Narcan) that has been diluted in normal saline to equal 10 ml until an adequate respiratory rate returns but pain relief remains intact.
    4. Give an intramuscular (IM) injection of 0.4 mg of naloxone (Narcan) that has been diluted in normal saline to equal 10 ml.

Copyright © 2004, Elsevier Science (USA). All Rights Reserved.

Supporting Sensory/Perceptual Function

PURPOSE

This chapter discusses key concepts that relate to the nursing diagnosis *Sensory/perceptual alteration* (visual, auditory, kinesthetic, gustatory, tactile, olfactory). It describes the normal physiology of sensation and perception, and a variety of factors affecting sensory/perceptual function.

MATCHING

1. ____ auditory
2. ____ gustatory
3. ____ kinesthetic
4. ____ olfactory
5. ____ ototoxic
6. ____ perception
7. ____ presbycusis
8. ____ presbyopia
9. ____ reticular activating system
10. ____ sensation
11. ____ sensory deprivation
12. ____ sensory overload
13. ____ tactile
14. ____ visual

a. the reception of stimulation through receptors of the nervous system

b. the conscious mental recognition or registration of a sensory stimulus, as, for example, when a person smells a sweet fragrance and gets a mental image of a cherry

c. having a damaging effect on cranial nerve VIII or the organs of hearing and balance

d. results from excessive environmental stimuli or a level of stimulus beyond the person's ability to absorb or comprehend it

e. located in the midbrain and thalamus; keeps the brain aroused

f. a decrease in the elasticity of the lens with age that impairs the ability to focus on near objects

g. a sensorineural hearing loss of high-frequency tones that occurs in the elderly and may lead to a loss of all hearing frequencies

h. pertaining to the sensation of sight

i. pertaining to the sensation of hearing

j. pertaining to the sensation of taste

k. pertaining to the sensation of touch

l. pertaining to the sensation of smell

m. pertaining to the sensation of position

n. inadequate reception or perception of environmental stimuli

TRUE OR FALSE

15. ____ Nurses observe sensory deficits more commonly in infants because of age-related changes in their sense organs.

16. ____ The cerebral cortex must be alerted or aroused to perceive and produce a conscious act in response to stimuli.

17. ____ Taste sensations decline normally with age.

18. ____ Adolescents are at risk for hearing loss if they are exposed to chronic loud noise.

19. ____ The Weber and Rinne tests are auditory screening tests used to evaluate the client for high-frequency hearing loss.

Copyright © 2004, Elsevier Science (USA). All Rights Reserved.

20. ____ Ageusia is the complete loss of taste.

21. ____ A hearing aid will not be damaged by x-ray examinations.

FILL-IN-THE-BLANKS

22. The human body has six types of _____ receptors, which pertain to sensations and sensory structures of the body.

23. _____ is commonly called crossed eyes and occurs in about 5% of children under the age of 4 years.

24. A _____ loss results from a problem in the outer and middle ear that reduces sensitivity to tones received by air conduction.

25. The sensation of smell declines with _____, nerve damage, or the presence of other odors in the nasal passages.

26. The _____ alphabet chart is used most commonly and appropriately for adults and older children to test their visual acuity.

27. Corneal _____ is indicated for diagnosis of corneal trauma, foreign bodies, corneal abrasions, or corneal ulcers.

28. The client hospitalized in an intensive care unit following major trauma or surgery is at risk for sensory _____.

EXERCISING YOUR CLINICAL JUDGMENT

29. Mrs. Pfannenstiel, the client from the chapter's case study, was most likely having difficulty doing which of the following things if she was scheduled for cataract surgery?
    1. Driving at night
    2. Selecting clothes that matched
    3. Reading a book since letters appeared small
    4. Reading a book because she had double vision

30. Mrs. Pfannenstiel was scheduled for cataract surgery. Which nursing diagnosis would be most appropriate?
    1. *Social isolation*
    2. *High risk for injury*
    3. *Disturbed sensory perception: visual*
    4. *Self-care deficit*

31. You instructed Mrs. Pfannenstiel to wear glasses, tape the metal shield over her operated eye at night, and not do heavy work, such as moving her furniture. Which nursing diagnosis would be most appropriate?
    1. *Social isolation*
    2. *Risk for injury*
    3. *Disturbed sensory perception: visual*
    4. *Self-care deficit*

TEST YOURSELF

32. Your client has double vision, which is also called:
    1. Presbyopia.
    2. Emmetropia.
    3. Diplopia.
    4. Ametropia.

33. Your elderly client has a hearing loss of high-frequency tones that may lead to a loss of all hearing frequencies. What type of hearing loss is this?
    1. Presbycusis
    2. Partial deafness
    3. Conductive loss
    4. Sensorineural

34. During your general assessment of your client's sensory/perceptual status, you asked your client if she was experiencing any numbness or tingling. Which of the following areas were you assessing?
    1. Hearing
    2. Sensation
    3. Vision
    4. Taste

35. You assessed bone conduction by placing the base of a vibrating tuning fork on the client's mastoid process and noting how many seconds passed before he could no longer hear it. Which of the following tests were you performing?
    1. Weber
    2. Rinne
    3. Whisper
    4. Finger-rubbing

36. Your 80-year-old client has had a progressive hearing loss over the past 8 months, has refused to participate in activities at the skilled nursing facility, and has often been found alone in his room. Which nursing diagnosis would be most appropriate?
    1. *Social isolation*
    2. *Altered thought processes*
    3. *Disturbed sensory perception: auditory*
    4. *Self-care deficit*

Copyright © 2004, Elsevier Science (USA). All Rights Reserved.

Supporting Verbal Communication

PURPOSE

This chapter introduces you to the physiological and behavioral concepts underlying *impaired verbal communication*. The chapter explores factors that affect communication and uses the nursing process as a framework for working with a client who has impaired verbal communication.

MATCHING

1. ____ aphasia

2. ____ articulation

3. ____ Broca's area

4. ____ communication

5. ____ dysarthria

6. ____ dysphagia

7. ____ dysphonia

8. ____ neologism

9. ____ paraphasia

10. ____ phonation

11. ____ resonance

12. ____ Wernicke's area

   a. difficulty swallowing

   b. a word substitution problem of the aphasic client who speaks fluently

   c. helps control the content of speech and affects auditory and visual comprehension

   d. the process of molding sounds into enunciated words and phrases

   e. the production of sound by the vibration of the vocal cords

   f. the forced vibration of a structure that is related to a source of sound and results in changes in the quality of the sound

   g. a complex process in which information is exchanged between two or more people

   h. difficulty producing vocal sounds

   i. a language disorder that results from brain damage or disease that involves speech centers in the brain

   j. the creation of words that are meaningless to the listener; a common language problem of the aphasic client

   k. the center of motor speech control

   l. impaired articulation

TRUE OR FALSE

13. ____ Vocal abuse, as from cheerleading, smoking, and alcohol abuse, can lead to laryngeal cancer, which may result in loss of the vocal folds and the ability to communicate verbally.

14. ____ Although verbal communication varies from culture to culture, nonverbal communication remains the same.

15. ____ A stimulating environment for a very young child aids in language acquisition.

16. ____ Communication is an important aspect of the nurse-client relationship.

17. ____ Self-concept plays a major role in communication patterns with other people.

18. ____ The use of a team approach is often necessary when working with a client who has impaired verbal communication.

19. ____ Active listening, when used with the client with impaired verbal communication, focuses

Copyright © 2004, Elsevier Science (USA). All Rights Reserved.

on the feelings of the client as well as nonverbal cues.

20. ____ Psychiatric illnesses do not affect communication with others.

21. ____ Self-talk involves talking about the activity as it is performed.

22. ____ When either the nurse or the client can speak the other person's language, but not fluently, they each know they are not at risk for misunderstanding the other.

FILL-IN-THE-BLANKS

23. Adult loss of language usually stems from _____ diseases.

24. _____ speech is telegram-like speech that lacks grammatical elements, such as articles, prepositions, and conjunctions.

25. When the client cannot comprehend spoken language and cannot articulate or write words, it is called _____ aphasia.

26. A disorder of voice volume, quality, or pitch, known as _____, can result from damage or disease of the larynx or vagus nerve.

27. A _____ is a temporary or permanent upper airway diversion that results in altered speech production.

28. The nurse should allow ample time for the client with _____ aphasia to respond verbally.

29. An alternative communication method for the client who has had a laryngectomy is the use of _____ speech, which involves eructation of swallowed air.

30. Limiting environmental stimuli and reducing distractions may increase comprehension in the client with _____ aphasia.

31. A client who is unable to communicate due to language barrier, and who has no one who can interpret is likely to have a nursing diagnosis of _____.

32. An endotracheal tube, tracheostomy, or tumor is considered a _____ barrier to communication.

EXERCISING YOUR CLINICAL JUDGMENT

Señor Martinez, the man identified in the chapter's case study, is a Mexican-American client who has tuberculosis, a communicable disease. You have been asked by the nurse who admitted this client to provide information needed to manage this health problem.

33. If you become concerned that Señor Martinez is responding "yes" to your questions without fully understanding them, you should:
    1. look for incongruity between the responses and the client's facial expressions.
    2. assume that he will answer the important questions correctly.
    3. ask the same question of his wife after the client answers.
    4. refrain from asking any further questions.

34. After obtaining an interpreter to assist with communication, you would direct your attention to which of the following individuals when obtaining information from Señor Martinez?
    1. The interpreter
    2. Señora Martinez
    3. Señor Martinez
    4. Attend equally to all three

35. If Señor Martinez speaks English to some extent, it would be most appropriate for you to communicate about which of the following before an interpreter becomes available?
    1. Reason for coming to the hospital
    2. Informed consent
    3. Reason for procedures
    4. Medication information

36. You would formulate which of the following expected outcomes for the nursing diagnosis of *Impaired verbal communication* for this client?
    1. Answers all questions correctly
    2. Expresses satisfaction with the communication process
    3. Provides nurse with sufficient information
    4. Adheres to instructions given while in the hospital

TEST YOURSELF

37. A nurse would assess the client with a tentative diagnosis of laryngitis for speech that is:
    1. hoarse or soft.
    2. spoken in a monotone.
    3. garbled.
    4. hesitant or deliberate.

38. A client is scheduled to have a tracheostomy performed. The nurse should make alternate plans for communication with this client:
    1. before the surgery is done.
    2. just after the client returns from surgery.
    3. on the day following surgery.
    4. as part of the discharge planning process.

Copyright © 2004, Elsevier Science (USA). All Rights Reserved.

39. The home health nurse notes that a client with the nursing diagnoses of *Impaired verbal communication* is frustrated about her ineffective communication skills and does not interact with family and friends as frequently as before. The nurse would tentatively make which of the following additional nursing diagnoses for this client?
    1. *Anxiety*
    2. *Powerlessness*
    3. *Impaired social interaction*
    4. *Altered role performance*

40. The nurse is communicating with a client who has Broca's aphasia. It would be most appropriate to do which of the following to enhance the client's ability to speak?
    1. Give directions in concise, quick, and sharp tones.
    2. Ask the client several questions at once so the client can formulate answers to all.
    3. Give lengthy, detailed explanations.
    4. Allow ample time for the client to respond to the nurse's communications.

41. The nurse is providing health teaching to adolescents about the risk of brain and spinal cord injuries, which often result in impaired verbal communication. The nurse would encourage these individuals to avoid using which of the following?
    1. Drugs and alcohol
    2. Seatbelts
    3. Helmets
    4. Protective sports equipment

Copyright © 2004, Elsevier Science (USA). All Rights Reserved.

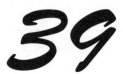

Managing Confusion

PURPOSE

This chapter explores factors that affect normal cognition and concepts that underlie *acute and chronic confusion*. It describes how to use the nursing process to work with the client experiencing either acute or chronic confusion.

MATCHING

1. ____ affect

2. ____ agnosia

3. ____ apraxia

4. ____ attention

5. ____ awareness

6. ____ cognition

7. ____ confusion

8. ____ consciousness

9. ____ delirium

10. ____ delusions

11. ____ dementia

12. ____ hallucinations

13. ____ judgment

14. ____ memory

15. ____ orientation

16. ____ pseudo-dementia

17. ____ sundown syndrome

a. the state of being awake and alert enough to react to stimuli; also called awareness

b. the retention or storage of information learned about the world

c. false personal beliefs

d. an awareness of person, place, and time

e. the observable expression of feelings or emotions; changes as chronic confusion progresses, as does the client's personality

f. the ability to focus on an object or activity

g. the failure to recognize or identify objects despite an intact sensory ability

h. depression that is misinterpreted as dementia

i. the state in which the individual experiences or is at risk of experiencing a disturbance in cognition, attention, memory, and orientation of an undetermined origin or onset

j. the process of knowing and interacting with the world; also called thought

k. involves multiple cognitive deficits including impairment of memory and judgment, and resulting in a progressive decline in intellectual functioning

l. the state of being awake and alert enough to react to stimuli; also called consciousness

m. sensory reactions in the absence of real stimuli

n. the inability to carry out motor activities despite the functional ability to perform them

o. a disturbance in consciousness or a change in cognition that develops over a short time

p. the ability to make rational decisions

q. a worsening of behavior that occurs as the sun goes down, especially after dark

TRUE OR FALSE

18. ____ Confusion is a condition that occurs only in the older adult.

19. ____ Acute confusion in the older adult usually develops over hours or days.

20. ____ Perceptual difficulties, such as illusions and hallucinations, may occur in acute confusion.

Copyright © 2004, Elsevier Science (USA). All Rights Reserved.

21. ____ Because cognitive changes occur more slowly with chronic confusion, the client does not lose the ability to judge his or her own safety.

22. ____ The loss of ability to perform activities of daily living occurs in the third stage of chronic confusion.

23. ____ Lack of an appropriate and complete mental status examination can be a barrier to identifying confusion.

24. ____ A child who develops a high fever is at risk for experiencing acute confusion.

25. ____ The nurse should not include attention span when conducting a mental status exam.

26. ____ Anxiety is a common client reaction in both acute and chronic confusion.

27. ____ The nurse should use pale muted colors or symbols used to identify the room of a client with chronic confusion.

FILL-IN-THE-BLANKS

28. Pick's disease is characterized by the formation of Pick's cells in the _____ and _____ lobes of the brain.

29. Cerebral hypoxia due to a medical condition can cause _____ confusion.

30. Acute confusion in the older adult typically occurs at _____.

31. A disrupted _____ rhythm is a classic symptom of acute confusion.

32. Dementia of the _____ type is the most common in older adults.

33. A person who cannot interpret proverbs during an assessment has a loss of _____ thinking.

34. A client who does not brush the hair due to lack of recall about the purpose of the hairbrush is said to have an _____.

35. Often an older adult will exhibit a change in mental status with a serious infection instead of a _____.

36. A client who can recall people and events from 30 years ago is said to have an intact _____ memory.

37. A client who is unaware of environmental hazards due to confusion may have the nursing diagnosis *Risk for* _____.

EXERCISING YOUR CLINICAL JUDGMENT

Mr. Tellis, the man identified in the chapter's case study, has a nursing diagnosis of *Acute confusion* related to disturbances in cerebral metabolism secondary to urinary tract infection as evidenced by agitation, inattention, and fluctuating consciousness. You have been assigned to work with Mr. Tellis on the day after hospital admission.

38. One of the expected outcomes formulated for Mr. Tellis in relation to this nursing diagnosis is "client will experience no injury." Which of the following actions would be most helpful in achieving this outcome?
    1. Restrict visitors as much as possible.
    2. Assist with ambulation and toileting as needed.
    3. Leave bed's side rails lowered at all times.
    4. Encourage him to stay in bed by obstructing the path to the bathroom with chairs.

39. Which of the following approaches to communicating with Mr. Tellis will be helpful in minimizing confusion and maintaining the client's dignity?
    1. Divide his care among several staff members.
    2. Give directions quickly and with a firm tone of voice.
    3. Focus on his real message and concerns during conversation.
    4. Quiz him about orientation level with each encounter.

40. Mr. Tellis lost most of his last night's sleep with the events surrounding admission. Which of the following strategies should be used to help reestablish his sleep-wake pattern?
    1. Schedule medications and care to allow for at least one uninterrupted 4-hour block of sleep each night.
    2. Make sure all visitors go home by at least 8 PM.
    3. Keep the door to his room open with the hall lights on.
    4. Encourage frequent naps during the day in case there are unexpected interruptions to sleep at night.

41. Mr. Tellis requires intermittent reorientation to his environment. Which of the following environmental cues would be most helpful?
    1. Bright lighting 24 hours a day
    2. No lighting during nighttime hours
    3. Name of caregivers written on a small pad on the night table
    4. Clock and calendar on wall at foot of bed

Copyright © 2004, Elsevier Science (USA). All Rights Reserved.

TEST YOURSELF

42. A nurse is conducting a mental status examination for a client newly immigrated to the United States. Which of the following questions, if asked by the nurse, would be least helpful in determining whether confusion is present?
    1. "What is your name?"
    2. "What did you eat for breakfast?"
    3. "Did any family members visit you today?"
    4. "Who was the first president of the United States?"

43. The nurse who is working with a client with chronic confusion would not assess which of the following factors?
    1. Impaired socialization
    2. A change in level of consciousness
    3. Long-standing cognitive impairment
    4. Altered response to stimuli

44. A client has been placed in a protective environment due to chronic confusion and irreversible dementia. The client has been disoriented to person, place, and time for at least 6 months. The nurse would choose which of the following most precise nursing diagnoses for this client?
    1. *Acute confusion*
    2. *Chronic confusion*
    3. *Impaired environmental interpretation syndrome*
    4. *Altered thought processes*

45. A nurse is caring for a client who seems confused, and lost a spouse 3 months ago. The nurse would determine that the client is experiencing feelings of depression more than confusion if the client:
    1. is worse in the morning than any other time of day.
    2. has visual hallucinations.
    3. is not preoccupied by certain people or events.
    4. does not exaggerate and is unaware of inabilities.

46. A confused client is hallucinating that someone is trying to steal the client's clothing in the closet. The nurse who is looking for a deeper meaning to this episode would pursue which of the following themes in conversation with this client?
    1. Money
    2. Safety
    3. Food
    4. Loneliness

Copyright © 2004, Elsevier Science (USA). All Rights Reserved.

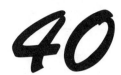

Promoting Self-Concept

PURPOSE

This chapter introduces you to self-concept, self-esteem, personal identity, role performance, and body image as they relate to clients. It provides direction in using the nursing process in caring for a client with an alteration in one or more of the components of self-concept.

MATCHING

1. ____ body image

2. ____ personal identity

3. ____ role

4. ____ role performance

5. ____ self-concept

6. ____ self-esteem

    a. a relatively enduring set of attitudes and beliefs about both the physical self and the psychological self

    b. includes the roles a person assumes or is given

    c. the organizing principle of the personality that accounts for the unity, continuity, consistency, and uniqueness of a person

    d. the degree to which a person has a positive evaluation of self based on perceptions of how one is viewed by others as well as view of the self

    e. a person's perception of his or her body

    f. a homogeneous set of behaviors, attitudes, beliefs, principles, and values that are normatively defined and expected of someone in a given social position or status in a group

TRUE OR FALSE

7. ____ Self-concept is not a static state but one that develops and changes over time.

8. ____ Low self-esteem can result in lack of confidence and inability to act in one's own best interest.

9. ____ According to Maslow, self-esteem develops before the need for belonging and being loved by others is met.

10. ____ Erikson describes the development of self-esteem in eight stages that correspond to a period in the life span.

11. ____ Research has demonstrated a negative correlation between positive self-esteem and positive health practices.

12. ____ An inability to perform role responsibilities can negatively affect other aspects of self-concept, especially self-esteem.

13. ____ Socioeconomic status has no relationship to self-concept.

14. ____ Loss of a spouse, good job, or previous good health can easily lower self-esteem.

15. ____ Fatigue, illness, and surgery are examples of physiological factors that can affect self-esteem.

16. ____ Nurses should conduct an in-depth assessment of self-concept with all clients.

FILL-IN-THE-BLANKS

17. The four components of self-concept are self-esteem, personal identity, role performance, and _____ _____.

18. At the top of Maslow's hierarchy of needs is _____ -_____.

19. According to Erikson's stages of development, adolescence involves development of _____.

20. The ability to influence and control others, according to Coopersmith, is termed _____ / _____.

Copyright © 2004, Elsevier Science (USA). All Rights Reserved.

21. The components of personal identity are
    _____, _____, and _____ images.

22. Self-esteem in infants and preschoolers can be
    related to the type of _____ a child receives.

23. Behaviors such as smoking, overeating, substance
    abuse, school difficulties, and early sexual
    experimentation can be associated with low
    _____ -_____.

24. The client's affective experience of the self,
    manifested as any negative self-feelings, is the
    defining characteristic for the nursing diagnosis of
    _____ _____ _____.

25. A sense of powerlessness can result in the nursing
    diagnosis of _____ *low self-esteem.*

26. If the client has a major change in body structure or
    function, the nurse should assess that client for the
    presence of the nursing diagnosis _____
    _____ _____.

EXERCISING YOUR CLINICAL JUDGMENT

Nancy Ward, the 43-year-old Navajo woman introduced
in the chapter's case study, has a disturbance in self
esteem due to a breast mass that requires biopsy. Recall
that Nancy's husband, who died 6 months ago from
complications of alcohol abuse, diabetes, and heart disease, abused her physically and emotionally during their
marriage. You see Nancy in the clinic when she comes to
receive the biopsy results.

27. If you were focusing on the influence of her
    husband's behavior on Nancy's self-concept,
    you might have selected which of the following
    alternate nursing diagnoses?
    1. *Situational low self-esteem*
    2. *Chronic low self-esteem*
    3. *Ineffective role performance*
    4. *Disturbed body image*

28. If you were to focus on how to promote Nancy's
    feelings of acceptance/worthiness as part of her
    self-esteem, you would include which of the
    following people in her care?
    1. Physician and nurse manager of the clinic
    2. Tribal medicine man (shaman) and friend that
       came to clinic with her
    3. Clinic social worker and billing clerk
    4. Radiologist and continuing care nurse from the
       affiliated hospital

29. Nancy is told by the physician that the breast
    mass is cancerous and that surgery will be
    needed. You would interact with Nancy,
    expecting that which of the following will be
    her first reaction?
    1. Shock and disbelief
    2. Anger
    3. Depression
    4. Acceptance

30. In trying to assist Nancy to adjust to the idea of the loss
    of a breast, you could inquire whether she is interested
    in talking to which of the following individuals?
    1. The surgeon who took the breast biopsy
    2. The pathologist who did the examination of the
       breast tissue
    3. Someone from Reach to Recovery who has lost
       a breast herself
    4. The staff who will be doing her preadmission
       testing before surgery

31. To foster a sense of power and control in Nancy
    about her upcoming surgery, you would use which
    of the following approaches?
    1. Remind Nancy that emotional healing is a
       matter of determination and courage.
    2. Tell her of the scheduled date for surgery as soon
       as it is known.
    3. Give her a list of instructions that must be
       followed before the surgery.
    4. Allow her to make as many decisions about the
       upcoming procedure as possible.

TEST YOURSELF

32. The nurse who is teaching a client with a new
    colostomy about colostomy care and management
    is indirectly increasing the client's sense of which
    of the following?
    1. Competence/mastery
    2. Power/control
    3. Moral worth/virtue
    4. Acceptance/worthiness

33. To reduce the impact of a recent loss on the client's
    self-concept, the nurse would assist the client to
    focus on which of the following?
    1. Past religious habits
    2. Personal successful coping skills
    3. The importance of forgetting negative events
    4. The negative attributes of the object of the loss

34. The nurse would look for other evidence of low self-
    esteem in a client who does which of the following?
    1. Accepts compliments with grace and ease
    2. Takes negative feedback from others in stride
    3. Continually seeks acceptance from others
    4. Is proud of personal accomplishments, but not
       boastful

Copyright © 2004, Elsevier Science (USA). All Rights Reserved.

35. The nurse would determine that which of the following clients is most at risk for developing issues with self-concept?
    1. A client who must take medication for allergies
    2. A client who gets short of breath after walking up two flights of stairs
    3. A client who has a gallbladder that must be removed
    4. A client who has suffered facial burns

36. A postoperative client who is also the mother of four is overexerting herself with housework and child-care responsibilities. In working with this client, the nurse incorporates the understanding that this client is experiencing a values conflict in which of the following areas of self-esteem?
    1. Competence/mastery
    2. Power/control
    3. Moral worth/virtue
    4. Acceptance/worthiness

37. The nurse is evaluating effects of an intervention on a client's self-concept. If the nurse were interested in using a subjective approach to evaluation, that nurse would select which of the following methods as most appropriate?
    1. The client's self-report of progress
    2. A standardized questionnaire
    3. A rating scale
    4. Observation of the client's behavior

Copyright © 2004, Elsevier Science (USA). All Rights Reserved.

Managing Anxiety

PURPOSE

This chapter introduces you to concepts of anxiety as they are manifested in the health care setting. It uses the nursing process as a framework for interacting with clients experiencing anxiety.

MATCHING

1. ____ adaptation

2. ____ anxiety

3. ____ anxiety disorder

4. ____ anxiolytics

5. ____ panic

6. ____ pathological anxiety

   a. a disorder that is accompanied by a relentless, ineffective mechanism designed to compel the person to lessen the supposed danger that is triggering the anxiety response

   b. variety of medications used to treat anxiety

   c. a disproportionate anxiety response to a given stimulus by virtue of its intensity or duration

   d. described as a diffuse, highly uncomfortable, sometimes vague sense of apprehension or dread accompanied by one or more physical sensations

   e. self-regulation of the whole person in relation to change

   f. a vivid, acute state of overwhelming fear with intense physiological, psychological, and behavioral symptoms

TRUE OR FALSE

7. ____ Anxiety is caused by interplay of factors that can be internal, external, or both.

8. ____ A person can actually create or worsen his or her own anxiety.

9. ____ When a client is in a state of panic, he or she may faint or freeze.

10. ____ Anxiety disorders are fairly uncommon in today's society due to the number of medications available.

11. ____ A phobia is a specific type of fear that is often exaggerated and incapacitating.

12. ____ A healthy lifestyle does not make us immune to stress, but may help us to weather it better.

13. ____ Learning theory suggests that anxiety is not a learned behavior.

14. ____ Cognitive characteristics of anxiety can include blocking of thoughts, forgetfulness, and impaired concentration or problem-solving ability.

15. ____ The nursing diagnosis of *Fear* is appropriate when the client has an intense feeling of dread related to an identifiable source that the client can verify.

16. ____ A panic attack is a gradual, discrete feeling of overpowering fright accompanied by physiological symptoms and thoughts of losing control, impending catastrophe, or death

FILL-IN-THE-BLANKS

17. Anxiety can be considered as falling into one of two primary categories, either a threat to _____ integrity or a threat to _____ integrity.

18. A core dynamic theme found at all levels of anxiety is a sense of _____.

19. In the level of anxiety that is _____, the person's perceptual field is completely distorted.

20. If anxiety impedes daily living and productivity, it is labeled as _____.

21. A client who has a persistent thought, image, or impulse that causes anxiety, and that the client cannot set aside, is said to have an _____.

Copyright © 2004, Elsevier Science (USA). All Rights Reserved.

22. _____ theory proposes that anxiety comes from unconscious conflicts that arose from real or symbolic events and situations that were threatening in infancy or childhood.

23. _____ is the nursing diagnosis that applies when the client believes that he or she has no control over situations or events.

24. Being admitted to a hospital can be considered to be an _____ factor that produces anxiety.

25. An _____-_____ disorder is marked by uncontrollable thoughts, images, or impulses and behavioral rituals that the client cannot dismiss.

26. Lack of access to health care services due to inadequate insurance is considered to be an _____ factor contributing to anxiety.

EXERCISING YOUR CLINICAL JUDGMENT

Ms. Adkins, the 42-year-old divorced woman introduced in the chapter's case study, has a history of cardiac disease and panic attacks. Her 16-year-old son told her before the onset of symptoms that he wishes to move in with his father. While she is being evaluated for a cardiac cause of chest pain, she is also given the nursing diagnosis *Anxiety* by the admitting nurse. You come on duty to relieve the admitting nurse and take over the care of Ms. Adkins.

27. Ms. Adkins tells you that she cannot convince her son to remain living in her home. She goes on to say that she feels that she has no control over her situation or life events. Based on these statements, you might also consider which of the following viable alternate nursing diagnoses for Ms. Adkins?
    1. *Sensory-perceptual alterations*
    2. *Powerlessness*
    3. *Fear*
    4. *Altered thought processes*

28. You identify a short-term goal with Ms. Adkins, which is to identify her own anxiety symptoms and participate in care planning. You determine that she has met the first expected outcome when she is able to:
    1. verbally identify signs and symptoms of escalating anxiety.
    2. sleep at least in 6-hour blocks.
    3. demonstrate relaxation techniques.
    4. use problem-solving skills.

29. While you are talking with Ms. Adkins, you try to "tune in" to the feelings behind her words. In this instance, you are using which of the following interventions to reduce anxiety?
    1. Communicating a sense of caring
    2. Giving permission
    3. Listening actively
    4. Modifying the environment

TEST YOURSELF

30. The nurse who is assessing for physiological evidence of anxiety in a client would look for:
    1. bradycardia.
    2. excessive salivation.
    3. constricted pupils.
    4. urinary frequency.

31. The nurse would formulate which of the following expected outcomes to measure whether a client has experienced a reduction in anxiety?
    1. Inability to use problem-solving skills
    2. Inability to identify stressors associated with anxiety
    3. Reduced tension, irritability, tremors, and sweating
    4. Lack of participation in decision making

32. The nurse who assesses energy fields and uses appropriate interventions to modulate and balance the energy field is using which of the following forms of complementary therapy?
    1. Relaxation
    2. Music therapy
    3. Spiritual support
    4. Touch therapy

Copyright © 2004, Elsevier Science (USA). All Rights Reserved.

42

Managing Vulnerability

PURPOSE

This chapter describes the domains of the Vulnerable Populations Conceptual Model. It identifies factors affecting vulnerability and describes the key components of assessing a vulnerable population. It also describes key interventions for the diagnoses of *Hopelessness* and *Powerlessness* in vulnerable populations.

MATCHING

1. ____ community diagnosis
2. ____ community health nursing
3. ____ epidemiology
4. ____ focus group
5. ____ health status
6. ____ human capital
7. ____ key informant
8. ____ opinion survey
9. ____ participant-observation
10. ____ parish nursing
11. ____ public health nursing
12. ____ relative risk
13. ____ resource availability
14. ____ social integration
15. ____ social status
16. ____ vulnerable populations
17. ____ windshield survey

a. ratio of the risk of poor health among populations who do not receive resources and are exposed to risk factors compared with those populations who do receive resources and are not exposed to these risk factors

b. field of nursing that promotes and preserves the health of populations

c. the practice of promoting and protecting the health of populations

d. the position of an individual in relation to others in the society

e. refers to the availability of socioeconomic and environmental resources

f. includes age- and gender-specific morbidity and mortality

g. a method of community assessment that examines formal and informal social systems at work

h. a registered nurse who is employed by (or volunteers) a religious or health care organization for the purpose of providing nursing care to members of a church congregation.

i. a diagnosis for a group or a community

j. social groups who have limited resources and consequently are at high risk for myriad health-related problems

k. a method of data collection in which the researcher drives through a neighborhood to conduct a general assessment of that neighborhood through observation

l. study of the cause and distribution of disease, disability, and death among groups of people

m. is a method of data collection in which 6 to 12 people from a group or aggregate are brought together for discussion, guided when necessary by a skilled, nonjudgmental leader

n. having a harmonious relationship with society in which the person participates as a full member of the society

o. includes income, jobs, education, and housing. Poverty, social inequality, poor educational resources and limited vocational resources are just a few of the socioeconomic constraints found in vulnerable populations

Copyright © 2004, Elsevier Science (USA). All Rights Reserved.

p. a community leader, professional, politician, or business person who possesses knowledge of the needs of the community and who can act as a useful source of data and a supporter of new programs

q. a method of data collection performed through telephone interviews, mailed questionnaires, door-to-door interviews, or at clinic sites

TRUE OR FALSE

18. _____Resource availability includes human capital, social integration, social status, and access to health care.

19. _____ For adolescent girls, the combination of high socioeconomic status, poor academic achievement, lack of available jobs, and the resultant feelings of low self-esteem may lead to pregnancy as the only reasonable alternative.

20. _____ For a person to have hope there must be a desire and some expectation that the desire will be fulfilled.

21. _____ A client who has a perception of power seeks knowledge and takes action to affect the outcome of the illness or to manage health.

22. _____ Hope cannot be present when the client feels no ability to control a situation.

23. _____ Both hope and power have to do with clients' ability to achieve goals.

24. _____ Only clients can empower themselves.

FILL-IN-THE-BLANKS

25. The Vulnerable Populations Conceptual Model provides a framework for understanding the relationships among the limited resource availability, the health-related _____ factors, and the _____ status of vulnerable populations.

26. Human capital includes income, jobs, education, and _____.

27. _____ _____ is reflected in power to control the political process and the distribution of resources.

28. _____ isolation is one of the well-known risks of elderly persons who live alone in the community.

29. Hope on the unconscious level is a life force that provides the _____ to drive the individual forward.

30. The primary distinction between *Hopelessness* and *Powerlessness* rests in the concept of _____.

31. To empower another individual you need to respect the individual's capacity for _____-_____.

EXERCISING YOUR CLINICAL JUDGMENT

Brenda Carter, referred to in this chapter's case study, is a single mother living alone with her 2-year-old child. She tells you, "I am just stuck here with this baby with no chance to do anything." She is socially isolated and has been in abusive relationships.

32. During your nursing assessment, you asked Brenda about her safety in her neighborhood. This would be an example of which type of needs assessment?
    1. Physical
    2. Psychological
    3. General
    4. Social

33. Brenda has broken off relations with her parents. She tells you she misses them. A potential nursing intervention would be to:
    1. acknowledge her parents' disappointment with her.
    2. help her contact her parents.
    3. encourage her to make a new life for herself and her baby.
    4. have her attend group counseling for pregnant teenagers.

34. You have been working with Brenda to help her deal with her feelings of hopelessness due to her parents refusing to allow her to return home. She says that they told her, "You wanted to be an adult, now act like one." Brenda was diagnosed as suffering from *Hopelessness*. A few weeks later she tells you that she has accepted living at the local home for unwed mothers and no longer feels hopeless about her situation. Your evaluation of *Hopelessness* may mean that she:
    1. needs to continue trying to win her parents back.
    2. has achieved acceptance of her situation, which cannot be changed at this time.
    3. should immediately be referred to mental health for counseling about her parents' rejection of her.
    4. is unrealistic about her situation.

TEST YOURSELF

35. Vulnerable social groups include which of the following?
    1. People subjected to intolerance, the poor, and those associated with a stigma
    2. Teenagers and people living in rural areas
    3. Infants and clients older than 60 years of age
    4. Those with resources, as well as children and the elderly

Copyright © 2004, Elsevier Science (USA). All Rights Reserved.

36. Your client has been diagnosed with breast cancer. She believes that through her own actions, behaviors, or personal characteristics she can affect her outcome. She feels in control of her situation. This is an example of which concept?
    1. "Power over"
    2. Human capital
    3. Hope
    4. Personal control

37. At the health department's teen clinic, adolescent girls and teen mothers are routinely screened for symptoms of conflict with their parents and with their partners. This is an example of which type of assessment of vulnerability?
    1. Hopelessness
    2. Physical needs
    3. Social needs
    4. Psychological needs

38. As a nurse, you can offer a client hope by:
    1. offering empathy or understanding of the client's feelings associated with being in a desolate situation.
    2. calling the mental health center and getting the client an appointment.
    3. referring the client to the public health department for follow-up care.
    4. telling the client to improve his or her self-esteem.

39. Your client has been diagnosed with diabetes. You can empower the client by:
    1. helping the client to develop, obtain, and use resources.
    2. calling the American Diabetes Association to obtain information for the client.
    3. referring the client to the outpatient diabetic program.
    4. waiting until the client requests help.

Copyright © 2004, Elsevier Science (USA). All Rights Reserved.

Managing Functional Limitations

PURPOSE

This chapter discusses key concepts related to rehabilitation, common conditions that require rehabilitative services, role changes following injury, and the roles of various members of the interdisciplinary team. It cites assessment tools that can be used for a person with a functional disability and major nursing diagnoses for a person with a spinal cord injury.

MATCHING

1. ____ activities of daily living

2. ____ chronic illness

3. ____ chronicity

4. ____ community reintegration

5. ____ functional limitations

6. ____ handicap

7. ____ impairment

8. ____ instrumental activities of daily living

9. ____ rehabilitation

a. the process of adaptation or recovery, through which an individual suffering from a disabling condition, whether temporary or irreversible, participates to regain or attempts to regain maximum function, independence, and restoration

b. difficulties people may experience in performing activities of daily living (ADLs) or instrumental activities of daily living (IADLs)

c. the basic activities usually performed in the course of a normal day in a person's life such as eating, toileting, dressing, bathing, or brushing the teeth

d. food preparation, housekeeping, laundry, transportation, using the telephone, shopping, and handling finances

e. limitations resulting from any one of a variety of conditions, whether related to disease, trauma, or birth defect

f. a disadvantage experienced by a person as a result of impairment that limits the person's "normal" function

g. all impairments or deviations from normal that have one or more of the following characteristics: are permanent; leave residual disability; are caused by a nonreversible pathological condition; require special training of the client for rehabilitation; or are expected to require a long period of supervision, observation, or care

h. a broad term that encompasses chronic illnesses, as well as disease or congenital defects, that permanently alter a person's previous health status

i. the return and acceptance of a disabled person as a participating member of the community

TRUE OR FALSE

10. ____ *Ineffective role performance* is the nursing diagnosis that applies when there is an adverse change in the way a person perceives or enacts a role.

11. ____ It is estimated that about 19% of the U.S. population has some form of disability.

12. ____ The Association of Rehabilitation Nurses (ARN) is the specialty organization for rehabilitation nurses.

13. ____ A prosthetist helps fit braces, orthoses, and adaptive equipment to assist with normal

Copyright © 2004, Elsevier Science (USA). All Rights Reserved.

movement and prevent secondary complications of corrective braces.

14. ____ Assisted living facilities provide interdisciplinary care to people who do not require hospitalization but whose needs for care exceed availability from informal community resources.

15. ____ Environmental factors that can affect ability and disability of clients with functional limitations include the person's living situation, workplace, or time spent in leisure activities.

16. ____ For a client who has functional limitations, you have primary responsibility for documentation of the overall health status and functional assessment.

17. ____ The client with sensory neglect may have minor neglect or be experiencing a more severe form, in which a body part, most often a paralyzed arm, is not recognized.

FILL-IN-THE-BLANKS

18. Disabilities can be a result of _____, chronic illness, congenital defect, or _____ _____.

19. Nurses who care for those with functional limitations become experts in _____ and psychosocial assessment, _____ and bladder management, _____ care, nutrition, behavior, teaching, and family participation.

20. Clients with long-term health alterations often use prayer as a _____ mechanism and look to God or another spiritual being as a source of comfort.

21. _____ living facilities combine shelter with other support services, such as meals, housekeeping, and personal care.

22. The _____ with _____ Act is a significant piece of legislation that advocates for those with disabilities.

23. The _____ _____ _____ (FIM) scale is one of the most reliable and valid tools for measuring functional status.

24. Goals in rehabilitation are aimed at _____ function and preventing _____.

EXERCISING YOUR CLINICAL JUDGMENT

25. Which type of health care professional would most likely assess the range of motion, mobility, strength, balance, and gait of Robert, the 18-year-old student referred to in this chapter's case study, who has a complete C5-6 spinal cord injury?
    1. Recreational therapist
    2. Physical therapist
    3. Rehabilitation nurse
    4. Occupational therapist

26. Robert receives respite care. What type of service does this represent?
    1. Help with home maintenance
    2. Comprehensive services requiring medical care that can be managed at home
    3. Assistance with personal care
    4. Temporary service enabling informal caregivers to take a break from their caregiving responsibilities

27. Robert is unable to perform most of the basic self-care activities such as feeding, bathing, and toileting. What nursing diagnosis would be appropriate?
    1. *Self-care deficit*
    2. *Impaired physical mobility*
    3. *Activity intolerance*
    4. *Risk for injury*

TEST YOURSELF

28. Which term is appropriate to describe the difficulties that your clients who have functional disabilities face with their physical challenges in performing activities of daily living?
    1. Impairment
    2. Functional limitations
    3. Chronicity
    4. Handicap

29. Your client receives assistance from homemaker services. What type of help does she receive?
    1. Help with home maintenance
    2. Comprehensive services requiring medical care that can be managed at home
    3. Assistance with personal care
    4. Temporary service enabling informal caregivers to take a break from their caregiving responsibilities

Copyright © 2004, Elsevier Science (USA). All Rights Reserved.

30. When your client's family is evaluating a nursing home for their frail, elderly family member, they ask the staff what infection control measures are enforced. This question helps to evaluate which area of a nursing home assessment?
    1. Social, educational, recreational, and religious activities
    2. Location
    3. Safety
    4. Living environment

31. Your client with hemiplegia as a result of a stroke has tactile impairments. Which nursing diagnosis would be most appropriate for the problems associated with tactile impairments?
    1. *Self-care deficit*
    2. *Impaired physical mobility*
    3. *Disturbed sensory perception*
    4. *Risk for injury*

32. Falls are a common problem among older adults with reduced functional capacity and a major factor contributing to dependence. Which nursing diagnosis would be appropriate?
    1. *Self-care deficit*
    2. *Impaired physical mobility*
    3. *Disturbed sensory perception*
    4. *Risk for injury*

Copyright © 2004, Elsevier Science (USA). All Rights Reserved.

Managing Loss

PURPOSE

This chapter discusses key concepts that relate to the nursing diagnoses of *Anticipatory grieving, Dysfunctional grieving,* and *Imminent death.* It describes a focused assessment of a dying client. It also discusses interventions to help the client and family feel understood and facilitate grief work.

MATCHING

1. ____ anger
2. ____ anticipatory grief
3. ____ bereavement
4. ____ code status
5. ____ denial
6. ____ disenfranchised grief
7. ____ dysfunctional grieving
8. ____ normal grief
9. ____ grief attack
10. ____ grief work
11. ____ hospice
12. ____ loss
13. ____ mourning
14. ____ palliative care
15. ____ searching
16. ____ selective attention
17. ____ sense of presence
18. ____ thanatology

a. to rob or have something of value removed and is traditionally defined as being deprived through death, such as a widow who is deprived by the death of her husband

b. discipline of study and research that deals with death and death-related topics

c. the act of choosing when and to whom a person will give attention regarding a loss and allow thoughts and feelings to enter the conscious mind

d. occurs as the denial and disbelief are replaced with the growing awareness of reality

e. an unexpected, involuntary resurgence of acute grief-related emotions and behaviors triggered by routine events and sometimes accompanied by uncontrollable crying or emotional display

f. a term used to identify the specific orders for a client regarding whether to begin resuscitative actions, and the extent of those actions, at the time of a cardiac or respiratory arrest

g. a nonthreatening, comforting perception by the bereaved of the deceased's presence

h. the effort by a grieving person to acknowledge the physical and psychological pain associated with bereavement and to integrate the loss into the future

i. encompasses a very diverse and unique set of emotions and responses

j. the extended, unsuccessful use of intellectual and emotional responses by which individuals, families, and communities attempt to work through the process of modifying self-concept based on the perception of loss

k. grief that lacks social acknowledgment, validation, and support for the bereaved

l. the term used to describe social and cultural acts and expressions used by a bereaved person to convey thoughts and feelings of sorrow

m. a philosophical concept of providing palliative or supportive care to dying persons in which the goal of care at or near the end of life is to accentuate living and enhance the quality of life

n. involves the intellectual and emotional responses and behaviors by which individuals, families, and communities attempt to work through the

Copyright © 2004, Elsevier Science (USA). All Rights Reserved.

process of modifying self-concept based on the perception of potential loss

o. the removal, change, or reduction in value of something valued or held dear and the feelings that result

p. refers to conscious and unconscious efforts by the bereaved to negate the reality of the loss through finding the deceased alive and well

q. is an intellectual process that does not alter reality but is used to help the person cope with the undesired reality

r. the active total care of patients whose disease is not responsive to curative treatment...where control of pain, of other symptoms and of psychological distress and spiritual distress is paramount

TRUE OR FALSE

19. ____ Mourning honors the dead and helps manage emptiness after death.

20. ____ Normal grieving can lead to lifelong problems and breakdowns in psychological and physical health.

21. ____ The ultimate loss a person faces is his own death.

22. ____ Normal anticipatory grief includes making plans for living after an ill person dies.

23. ____ Until the reality of the loss has been acknowledged, further grief work is constrained.

24. ____ Seldom do people have feelings of relief or emancipation from burdens after a person's death.

25. ____ If you are comfortable facing the reality of your own death, you will find it difficult to provide support to others facing these same circumstances and issues.

FILL-IN-THE-BLANKS

26. Acts of mourning include _____ rituals, expressions of _____, and _____ practices.

27. The loss of _____ is recognized as the ultimate loss.

28. Cultural and societal mores commonly govern the behavioral responses associated with the _____ phase of grieving.

29. During the _____ phase the mind comes to clearly understand that the loss is irreversible and life has changed irrevocably.

30. When planning care for a terminally ill client, you are really caring for two clients, the dying person and the immediate _____ unit.

31. The most important intervention during the recognition: shock and denial phase of grief may be simply your _____.

32. _____ by other nurses or health care team members about attachments and feelings for clients in your care is detrimental both to you and to team dynamics.

EXERCISING YOUR CLINICAL JUDGMENT

33. Mr. Hashimoto, the 54-year-old first-generation Japanese-American client who was referred to in this chapter's case study, died with his family by his side. After his death his wife became nauseated, had abdominal cramping, and vomited. She felt heart palpitations and had trouble swallowing. She was in which phase of the grieving process?
    1. Dysfunctional grieving
    2. Recognition: shock and denial
    3. Reflection: physical, emotional, and spiritual suffering
    4. Redirection: reorganizing and moving forward

34. Mr. Hashimoto did not talk to staff about his loss because he felt that they were not receptive to his concerns. This is an example of which type of cognitive denial?
    1. Selective attention
    2. Deception
    3. True denial
    4. Anger

35. A year after Mr. Hashimoto's death, Mrs. Hashimoto continues to experience periods of acute grief-related emotions and behaviors triggered by routine events and sometimes accompanied by uncontrollable crying or emotional display. Which type of psychological response is she experiencing?
    1. Sense of presence
    2. Intrusive memories
    3. Grief attacks
    4. Dysfunctional grief

TEST YOURSELF

36. Nurses wore a black band on their nurses' caps at the time of Florence Nightingale's death. This is an example of what?
    1. Bereavement
    2. Mourning
    3. Loss
    4. Grief

Copyright © 2004, Elsevier Science (USA). All Rights Reserved.

37. This phase of the grief reaction has been called the "listen now, hear later" phase because it grants the grieving person time to buffer the truth while mobilizing coping resources to face the truth of a loss.
    1. Reflection: physical, emotional, and spiritual suffering
    2. Anticipatory grieving
    3. Recognition: shock and denial
    4. Redirection: reorganization and moving ahead

38. Sometimes a person develops physical symptoms experienced earlier by the deceased person, especially pains or specific somatic symptoms associated with the death. This is an example of which type of dysfunctional grief?
    1. Chronic
    2. Delayed
    3. Exaggerated
    4. Masked

39. Meeting the client's physical needs promptly, scheduling pain medications so they are being delivered to the client at the exact administration times, and touching and talking to the dying person are interventions to promote healthy grieving during which phase?
    1. Reflection: physical, emotional, and spiritual suffering
    2. Anticipatory grieving
    3. Recognition: shock and denial
    4. Redirection: reorganization and moving ahead

Copyright © 2004, Elsevier Science (USA). All Rights Reserved.

45

Maintaining Sexual Health

PURPOSE

This chapter discusses key concepts that relate to the nursing diagnoses *Ineffective sexuality patterns* and *Sexual dysfunction*. It discusses general concepts and the biological, psychological, social, and cultural influences on development of sexuality. It also describes issues in the health care of lesbian women and gay men.

MATCHING

1. ____ androgyny
2. ____ arousal
3. ____ bisexual
4. ____ gender
5. ____ gender identity
6. ____ gender role
7. ____ heterosexual
8. ____ homophobia
9. ____ homosexual
10. ____ libido
11. ____ orgasm
12. ____ sexual desire
13. ____ sexual dysfunction
14. ____ sexual identity
15. ____ sexuality
16. ____ sexual orientation
17. ____ sexual patterns

a. the state or quality of being sexual, including the collective characteristics that distinguish male and female

b. refers to a person's sex, either male or female

c. may be referred to as sexual identity, which is the internal belief or sense that one is male or female

d. may be referred to as gender identity, which is the internal belief or sense that one is male or female

e. refers to the outward appearance, behaviors, attitudes, and feelings deemed appropriate for males and females

f. an anthropological term; means that a person may display both male and female characteristics and may relate to both a male and female gender identity and role

g. refers to a person's sexual attraction and feelings of erotic potential toward a partner or toward members of either sex

h. type of sexual orientation in which one is attracted to members of the opposite gender

i. type of sexual orientation in which one is attracted to members of the same gender

j. type of sexual orientation in which one may be attracted to members of either gender

k. person's chosen expressions of sexuality

l. a wish to participate in sexual intimacy that is activated by thoughts, fantasies, emotions, and psychological wants and needs

m. physical and emotional stimuli heighten desire and begin the physiological changes that mark the sexual response cycle

n. a highly pleasurable involuntary response in which the clitoris, vagina, and uterus of the female or the penis of the male undergoes repeated muscular contractions

o. the conscious or unconscious sex drive or desire to pleasure or satisfy

p. implies a change or disruption in sexual health or function that the affected person views as unrewarding or inadequate

q. a fear of becoming homosexual through contact with lesbians and gay men or of having close or intimate feelings toward someone of the same sex

Copyright © 2004, Elsevier Science (USA). All Rights Reserved.

TRUE OR FALSE

18. ____ Puberty is a physiologically stressful time.

19. ____ Gender identity is an external belief that one is either male or female.

20. ____ Sexual patterns generally fit with the prevailing expectations of a particular culture or society.

21. ____ A characteristic of being sexually healthy includes a person's willingness to make adjustments in sexual functioning when limitations of illness, injury, unavailability of a partner, or other situations occur.

22. ____ Nurses routinely discuss their client's sexual health and concerns.

23. ____ Numerous health problems can have a biochemical effect on sexual energy and the ability to engage in sex.

24. ____ It is a myth that it is best for a man to be on the bottom during sex after a heart attack.

FILL-IN-THE-BLANKS

25. A person's sexuality is a vital component of health and is influenced by _____, psychological, social, and _____ forces.

26. Awareness of sexual feelings usually does not occur until _____, at the onset of mature sexuality.

27. _____ is a highly pleasurable involuntary response in which the clitoris, vagina, and uterus of the female or the penis of the male undergoes repeated muscular contractions.

28. The World Health Organization describes sexual health as the integration of somatic, _____, intellectual, and social aspects of sexual being in ways that are enriching and that enhance personality, communication, and _____.

29. Your anxiety and _____ in discussing sexual concerns will be communicated to your client.

30. A vital part of your assessment of a client with altered sexuality patterns is to understand the client's _____ knowledge and attitudes.

31. You should encourage children to tell a parent, teacher, or other trusted adult when a _____ is uncomfortable for them.

EXERCISING YOUR CLINICAL JUDGMENT

32. Lisa Simelli, the 46-year-old client from this chapter's case study who was diagnosed with breast cancer, expresses general concern regarding her sexuality. Which of the following nursing diagnoses would be most appropriate?
    1. *Ineffective sexuality patterns*
    2. *Sexual dysfunction*
    3. *Ineffective individual coping*
    4. *Hopelessness*

33. Ms. Simelli states that she is feeling unattractive and expresses concern about the results of her biopsy. In addition, she reports she has had no intercourse with her husband for the past 3 months. With this expanded data base of information, which of the following nursing diagnoses might the nurse also consider?
    1. *Ineffective sexuality patterns*
    2. *Sexual dysfunction*
    3. *Ineffective individual coping*
    4. *Hopelessness*

34. Ms. Simelli is fearful of disclosing her personal anxieties and beliefs about sex. You assure her that sometimes sharing personal information is necessary to provide the best possible health care. This is an example of which step of the PLISSIT model?
    1. Permission
    2. Limited information
    3. Specific suggestions
    4. Intensive therapy

TEST YOURSELF

35. Gender roles (e.g., whether a wife is encouraged to cut the wood for the fireplace), refer to which of the following?
    1. Outward appearance, behaviors, attitudes, and feelings deemed appropriate for males and females
    2. Internal belief that one is male or female
    3. Awareness and feelings of being male or female
    4. A person's chosen expressions of sexuality

36. During which phase of the sexual response cycle does a male experience the following: the head of the penis enlarges slightly, the scrotum thickens further and tenses, and two or three drops of preorgasmic fluid emerge from the head of the penis?
    1. Excitement
    2. Plateau
    3. Orgasm
    4. Resolution

Copyright © 2004, Elsevier Science (USA). All Rights Reserved.

37. Your client was raised to think that sexual intercourse is disgusting and dirty. This is an example of what kind of factor that affects sexuality?
    1. Developmental
    2. Psychological
    3. Physiological
    4. Psychiatric disorder

38. After your client had heart surgery, what advice would you give him about maintaining his sexual patterns?
    1. "It is best for you to be on the bottom during sex."
    2. "Impotence and lack of sex drive always occur after a heart attack."
    3. "If angina occurs during sex, you should permanently stop having sex."
    4. "You can safely resume sex within a few weeks or as soon as you feel ready."

39. Your client, a 12-year-old boy, masturbates. His minister says that masturbation is sinful. He is concerned that he is not normal. Which of the following nursing diagnoses would be most appropriate?
    1. *Ineffective sexuality patterns*
    2. *Sexual dysfunction*
    3. *Ineffective individual coping*
    4. *Hopelessness*

Copyright © 2004, Elsevier Science (USA). All Rights Reserved.

46

Supporting Stress Tolerance and Coping

PURPOSE

This chapter introduces you to the concepts of physiological and psychological stress, and the factors affecting one's ability to cope with stress. It provides guidelines on using the nursing process to work effectively with clients who are experiencing stress in their lives.

MATCHING

1. ____ adaptation
2. ____ adaptive coping
3. ____ anxiety
4. ____ compensating
5. ____ coping
6. ____ crisis
7. ____ defense mechanisms
8. ____ developmental crisis
9. ____ focusing
10. ____ homeostasis
11. ____ maladaptive coping
12. ____ psychoneuro-immunology
13. ____ reconstructing
14. ____ resilience
15. ____ situational crisis
16. ____ stress
17. ____ stressor

   a. the study of the interface between the brain and immunology

   b. tendency of biological systems to maintain relatively constant conditions in the internal environ-ment, while continuously interacting with and adjusting to changes originating within or outside the system

   c. mental processes used, without planning or even full awareness, to protect or defend one's (psychological) self from stress and maintain psychological homeostasis

   d. an individual's ability to recover from or successfully cope with both internal and external stresses

   e. a physiological response produced by the normal wear and tear of bodily processes and external and internal demands

   f. a physically or psychologically hazardous situation that is not easily anticipated and for which a person is inadequately prepared

   g. any effort directed toward management of dangerous, threatening, or challenging situations

   h. the description of a stress-causing agent

   i. an upset in a balanced or stable state for which the usual methods of adaptation and coping are not sufficient

   j. occurs when a person is unable to complete the tasks needed for a particular developmental level

   k. is a vague, uneasy feeling, the source of which is often nonspecific or unknown to the individual.

   l. works most effectively with stressors that cannot be avoided, such as illness, impending divorce, unexpected death, or the loss of a loved one

   m. process through which individuals accommodate changes in the internal or external environment to preserve functioning and pursue goals

   n. asking the client to focus on recognizing bodily signals that stress is interfering with comfort

Copyright © 2004, Elsevier Science (USA). All Rights Reserved.

o. feelings and behavior that decrease the quality of life and lead to unhealthy outcomes

p. a process that fosters problem solving, growth and development, and the ability to perceive reality and respond in a way that supports emotional and physical well-being

q. can enhance resilience by reconstructing stressful situations in a way that puts the experience in perspective

TRUE OR FALSE

18. ____ Stress results from attempts to balance internal and external environmental demands.

19. ____ In the resistance stage of the physiological stress response, the body cannot function defensively against the stressor.

20. ____ Lack of unconditional love can precipitate a developmental crisis in an infant.

21. ____ Sublimation involves using an excuse to justify behavior while disguising an unconscious motive.

22. ____ When assessing for stress tolerance and coping, it is helpful to ask clients if they are worrying about anything.

23. ____ Stress can cause some diseases and exacerbate others.

24. ____ What is stressful for one person in almost all cases is also stressful for another.

25. ____ Compensation is acting toward a stranger as if he or she were a significant other.

26. ____ Although all people react uniquely to stress, some have more reserve or capacity to resist challenges to self-integrity.

FILL-IN-THE-BLANKS

27. The first stage of the physiological stress response is the _____ _____ stage.

28. A person in _____ is faced with overwhelming adaptive tasks.

29. There are two major types of crises: _____ and _____.

30. A person who attributes unacceptable thoughts or feelings to others is using the defense mechanism of _____.

31. How a person tolerates and copes with stress is influenced by _____, lifestyle, culture, _____ _____, physiological characteristics, and psychological traits.

32. The _____ nervous system activity increases heart rate, cardiac output, respiratory rate, muscle tension, mental alertness, and glucose levels during a stressful event.

33. Both anxiety- and crisis-provoking situations challenge a person's _____ skills.

34. An inability to have children is generally considered a developmental crisis of _____.

35. At certain stages of coping, _____ is a useful and healthy defense mechanism that permits the client to retain hope and allows the individual to organize more effective ways of adapting to a stressful event.

EXERCISING YOUR CLINICAL JUDGMENT

Billy Osceola, the Native American of the Seminole tribe identified in the chapter's case study, is diabetic, drinks alcohol, and has developed signs of stump infection following a recent left below-knee amputation. He was using a special herbal concoction made by the tribe's medicine man to treat the painful stump area. After resisting attempts by a home health nurse to work with him in his home, he is ultimately readmitted to the hospital for treatment of the infection. You are now assigned to Mr. Osceola's care.

36. Based on your knowledge of Mr. Osceola thus far, you would select which of the following nursing diagnoses as most appropriate for him at this time?
    1. *Altered thought processes*
    2. *Ineffective denial*
    3. *Ineffective family coping*
    4. *Anxiety*

37. As a first step to assisting Mr. Osceola work through the stress of the amputation and its consequences, you would try to:
    1. confront his denial of the infection before admission.
    2. get a consult with a psychiatrist.
    3. establish a therapeutic relationship.
    4. make him identify past coping strategies.

38. If you wish to help Mr. Osceola cope by helping him gain control through knowledge, you would focus on teaching him:
    1. relaxation and deep breathing techniques.
    2. the relationship of his diabetes and drinking to the surgery he just had.
    3. that the medicine man, or shaman, is not very helpful in matters such as these.
    4. how to prevent further infection, control diabetes, and increase mobility.

Copyright © 2004, Elsevier Science (USA). All Rights Reserved.

39. Mr. Osceola shares with you that he finds comfort in listening to tribal music, especially the beat of the drums. Using knowledge of various coping methods, you would teach and encourage him to use which of the following while listening to this music?
    1. Relaxation
    2. Adaptive thinking
    3. Self-suggestion
    4. Coping thoughts

TEST YOURSELF

40. A coping method that is not conducive to alleviating stress in a healthy way would be:
    1. listening to music.
    2. overeating.
    3. talking to others about the stressor.
    4. crying or singing as an emotional release.

41. When working with a client experiencing a major stressor, the nurse would protect the client's "vulnerable self" by doing which of the following?
    1. Immediately break down any denial.
    2. Enlist the help of the client's social supports.
    3. Help the client identify inner strengths that can be used in this situation.
    4. Tell the client about the negative physiological effects of stress.

42. The nurse who is teaching relaxation techniques to a client would most likely incorporate which of the following methods in discussions with the client?
    1. Deep breathing and guided imagery
    2. Self-suggestion and coping thoughts
    3. Coping thoughts and inner dialog
    4. Adaptive thinking and self-suggestion

43. A client under extreme stress has come to the emergency room expressing thoughts of suicide. The nurse should take which of the following most appropriate actions?
    1. Locate and obtain resources to help with the crisis.
    2. Document the findings and then discharge the client to home.
    3. Encourage the client to resume antidepressant medications.
    4. Leave the client alone in a room to provide opportunity for reflective thought.

Copyright © 2004, Elsevier Science (USA). All Rights Reserved.

47

Supporting Family Coping

PURPOSE

This chapter describes the concepts of family, family function, family relationships, and caregiving. Family assessment criteria are identified as well as factors affecting an individual's ability to provide care family coping. The chapter provides potential nursing diagnoses that may be appropriate for family coping and caregiving. It provides goal-directed interventions to prevent or correct family problems and *Caregiver role strain*

MATCHING

1. ____ caregiver
2. ____ caregiver burden
3. ____ caregiver burnout
4. ____ caregiver stress
5. ____ caring
6. ____ closed system
7. ____ coping patterns
8. ____ extended family
9. ____ family
10. ____ family-centered nursing
11. ____ family dynamics
12. ____ intergenerational family
13. ____ nuclear family
14. ____ objective caregiver burden
15. ____ open system
16. ____ role conflict
17. ____ role stress
18. ____ single-parent family
19. ____ subjective caregiver burden
20. ____ system

a. unit includes the nuclear family as well as other relatives such as aunts, uncles, cousins, and grandparents who are committed to maintaining family ties

b. a set of integrated, interacting parts that function as a whole, with structure and patterns of function that accomplish the work of the whole

c. an emotion that occurs when a person has difficulty meeting the demands of a role

d. health care that focuses on the health of the family as a unit, as well as the maintenance and improvement in the health and growth of each person in that unit

e. exchanges matter, energy, and information with other systems and with the environment

f. households in which the children live with one parent, usually because of divorce, out-of-wedlock births, or the death of a spouse

g. a depletion of physical and mental energy caused by providing care for a chronically ill person over a long period

h. more than one generation of a family living together in one residence or within a small geographical area

i. two or more people united by a common goal to create a physical, cultural, spiritual, and nurturing bond

j. refers to the visible, tangible costs to the caregiver as measured in required behaviors or disruptions

k. one who provides care to a dependent or partially dependent family member or friend

l. incompatible expectations for behavior within a role, between two or more roles, or when a role is incongruent with a person's beliefs and values

m. composed of a husband, a wife, and their child/children living in a common household with one or both spouses gainfully employed

Copyright © 2004, Elsevier Science (USA). All Rights Reserved.

n. refers to strain or load borne by a family member who cares for an elderly, chronically ill, or disabled family member

o. refers to the caregiver's personal appraisal of a caregiving situation and the extent to which the person perceives it to be a burden

p. a set of integrated interacting parts that function as a whole and do not interact with other systems or the environment

q. the specific protective behaviors used by an individual or a family to respond to stressful situations

r. the ever changing pattern of interaction among family members; it is the forces at work within the family that create patterns of behavior.

s. a behavior of having regard for, cherishing, protecting, being responsible for, or attending to needs of others

t. refers to the caregiver's reaction to physical, emotional, sociocultural, financial, and environmental stressors brought on by the caregiving experience

TRUE OR FALSE

21. ____ The family is the basic social unit of society and has needs as a unit.

22. ____ The healthy family is an open system with complex interactions both within the family and in the external world.

23. ____ An unhealthy family will show genuine interest in learning to help the client.

24. ____ The family may or may not recognize that their coping is compromised.

25. ____ An appropriate nursing intervention to establish a nurse–family relationship is active listening.

26. ____ Interventions provided when a family is stressed or not focused are more easily remembered and accepted.

27. ____ *Caregiver role strain* may be increased—erase increased and change to minimized when the recipient and the caregiver predetermine how and by whom the care will be provided.

28. ____ Caregivers are more likely to experience *Caregiver role strain* when they have adequate support systems.

29. ____ An example of a cue that a family is at risk for *Caregiver role strain* is resurfacing of childhood issues with siblings.

30. ____ Financial costs associated with caregiving can cause many families to experience financial difficulties.

FILL-IN-THE-BLANKS

31. You will have to assess the needs of the _____ as well as the ill family member.

32. The primary functions of a family include the_____, _____ and social placement, reproductive, economic, and _____ care function.

33. Family _____ is the family unit's method of managing the stressors of family life.

34. Your first visit to the family is definitive in establishing a _____ relationship.

35. In many cases, caregivers enter their roles with _____ feelings.

36. Caregiver _____ refers to the caregiver's reaction to physical, emotional, sociocultural, financial, and environmental stressors brought on by the caregiving experience.

37. The caregiver's _____ of the burden, rather than the perception of other family members or health care providers, determines the impact on his or her life

38. Many caregivers do not have _____ into the role responsibilities involved in the day-to-day care of a dependent care receiver.

EXERCISING YOUR CLINICAL JUDGMENT

39. Mrs. Roddy's daughter, the client referred to in this chapter's case study, quits work to care for her ill mother. As a result, she experiences a financial hardship. Her stress originates from which one of the following sources?
    1. Interfamily
    2. Extrafamily
    3. Intrafamily
    4. Community

Copyright © 2004, Elsevier Science (USA). All Rights Reserved.

40. Mrs. Roddy is deteriorating physically and mentally. She is currently hospitalized, but her daughter insists that she be discharged to her home as opposed to a skilled nursing facility. The daughter is going to have to learn how to care for her mother's tracheostomy, gastrostomy tube feedings, Foley catheter, heparin lock, and multiple medications. Her daughter is currently:
    1. at *Risk for caregiver role strain.*
    2. experiencing *Caregiver role strain.*
    3. at *Risk for injury.*
    4. experiencing *Ineffective management of therapeutic regimen.*

41. As a home health nurse, you develop a plan of care with Mrs. Roddy's daughter that includes having a home health aide bathe Mrs. Roddy three times a week. This is an example of which nursing intervention?
    1. Engaging the assistance of family and friends
    2. Encouraging social support
    3. Setting realistic goals
    4. Providing direct assistance

TEST YOURSELF

42. Your client who is ill has a very supportive family. This is an example of which family function?
    1. Health care
    2. Socialization
    3. Affective
    4. Cognitive

43. The husband and wife could not agree on whose responsibility it was to clean their house. The husband believed it was his wife's responsibility to do the house cleaning, and his wife believed that the household duties should be shared. They are experiencing which one of the following stressors?
    1. Developmental stress
    2. Economic stress
    3. Role stress
    4. Role conflict

44. Your client is interested in learning about a low-salt diet. Both he and his wife have hypertension and want to change their eating habits. The most appropriate nursing diagnosis would be which of the following?
    1. *Impaired parenting*
    2. *Readiness for enhanced family coping*
    3. *Compromised family coping*
    4. *Disabled family coping*

45. A client, 80, has been living with her middle-aged son and his wife, who have been providing financial and emotional support. The relationship has been mutually satisfying and beneficial. Unfortunately, the client fell and fractured her hip. The family does not know how to manage the client's care. Which nursing diagnosis would be most appropriate?
    1. *Impaired parenting*
    2. *Readiness for enhanced family coping*
    3. *Compromised family coping*
    4. *Disabled family coping*

46. Your client is experiencing caregiver burnout. What is the recommended nursing intervention?
    1. Have her and the ill family member placed in a skilled nursing facility.
    2. Help her recognize her unrealistic expectation of herself and get respite care.
    3. Have her and the ill family member placed in assisted living facility for respite care.
    4. Help her recognize that she is experiencing burnout, then proceed with nursing intervention.

47. You praise your client's family caregiver for doing a good job in taking care of the client. This is an example of what type of nursing intervention to reduce *Caregiver role strain?*
    1. Promoting a realistic appraisal
    2. Allowing the client to ventilate
    3. Providing direct care
    4. Providing empathy

Copyright © 2004, Elsevier Science (USA). All Rights Reserved.

Supporting Spirituality

PURPOSE

This chapter discusses key concepts that relate to the nursing diagnoses *Spiritual distress, Risk for spiritual distress,* and *Readiness for enhanced spiritual well-being.* It discusses the concepts of spirituality, religion, and faith with the idea of providing spiritual care in nursing.

MATCHING

1. ____ agnostic
2. ____ atheist
3. ____ faith
4. ____ hope
5. ____ monotheism
6. ____ polytheism
7. ____ religion
8. ____ spiritual distress
9. ____ spirituality
10. ____ spiritual well-being

a. the experiences and expressions of one's spirit in a unique and dynamic process reflecting faith in God or a supreme being; connectedness with oneself, others, nature, or God; and integration of the dimensions of mind, body, and spirit

b. a belief system, including dogma, rituals, and traditions

c. the belief in the existence of one god who created and rules the universe

d. the belief in more than one god

e. a person who believes there is no God or a supreme being

f. a person who is undecided about the existence of God or a supreme being

g. belief in or commitment to something or someone greater than the self that helps a person realize purpose

h. the process of being and becoming by reflecting one's spirituality; it represents the totality of a person's inner resources, the wholeness of spirit and unifying dimension, a process of transcendence, and the perception of life as having meaning

i. an interpersonal process created through trust and nurtured by a trusting relationship with others, including God

j. a disruption that pervades the entire being and that integrates and transcends biological and social nature resulting in anguish of the human spirit

TRUE OR FALSE

11. ____ Religion can mean a social institution in which people participate together, rather than an individual searching alone for meaning in life.

12. ____ Spiritual and religious expressions are synonymous.

13. ____ By definition, faith is belief with proof. Each person chooses what to believe.

14. ____ Several research studies confirm that nurses commonly address spirituality.

15. ____ The fundamental teachings of Judaism are grouped around the concept of monotheism.

16. ____ Children do not have spiritual crises in the same sense as adults.

17. ____ Clients who despair or feel hopeless are more likely to die, or die sooner, even when there is little physiological disease to justify the death.

FILL-IN-THE-BLANKS

18. Religion can be viewed as a service to _____, organized within a specified set of beliefs and practices.

Copyright © 2004, Elsevier Science (USA). All Rights Reserved.

19. _____ is belief, expectancy, or trust that things will be better.

20. _____ believe in three gods, including the originator Lao Tzu.

21. Protestant churches have many ____ with a variety of differing beliefs.

22. All religious _____ and practices are bound to the culture and guide the group's lifestyle.

23. Clients who are experiencing a crisis are susceptible to _____ distress.

24. Many clients use _____ as an effective coping strategy for dealing with health crises.

EXERCISING YOUR CLINICAL JUDGMENT

25. Mr. Groves, the 56-year-old Mexican-American client from this chapter's case study, states that he is going to ask his priest why God causes diseases like cancer. You ask him if his wife is going to be present when he discusses his feelings with the priest. You tell him that you think he might be able to express himself more openly if his wife was not present during his conversation with the priest. What were you taking into consideration during your discussion with Mr. Groves?
    1. His religion
    2. His culture
    3. His family
    4. His psychological well-being

26. You ask Mr. Groves what has bothered him most about being sick. This is an example of which element of a spiritual assessment?
    1. To determine a client's beliefs, values, and concept of God or divine being
    2. To determine a client's sources of hope and strength
    3. To determine a client's religious practices
    4. To determine a client's perceived relationship between spiritual beliefs and health

27. If the expected outcome for Mr. Groves is to establish a meaningful relationship with himself, God, and others, the most likely nursing diagnosis is which of the following?
    1. *Ineffective individual coping*
    2. *Readiness for enhanced spiritual well-being*
    3. *Risk for spiritual distress*
    4. *Spiritual distress*

TEST YOURSELF

28. Activities such as prayer and going to church are examples of which characteristic of spirituality?
    1. General
    2. Being
    3. Knowing
    4. Doing

29. A person who is undecided about the existence of God or a supreme being is which of the following?
    1. An atheist
    2. A polytheist
    3. A monotheist
    4. An agnostic

30. Which nursing theorist stated that one assumption about the healing process is the premise that human nature is rooted in relatedness to the absolute truth of the creator?
    1. Watson
    2. Roy
    3. Travelbee
    4. Newman

31. If you help your client examine his or her life experiences to discover new meanings or reconnect to forgotten moments that represent significant meaning, which nursing intervention are you using?
    1. Life review
    2. Reminiscence
    3. Counseling
    4. Visualization

32. Your client who recently lost her infant expresses disbelief in God. Which nursing diagnosis would be most appropriate?
    1. *Ineffective individual coping*
    2. *Readiness for enhanced spiritual well-being*
    3. *Risk for spiritual distress*
    4. *Spiritual distress*

Copyright © 2004, Elsevier Science (USA). All Rights Reserved.

The Surgical Client

PURPOSE

This chapter describes the perioperative phases and factors that affect the surgical experience for a client. It discusses how you can use the nursing process to care for a client before, during, and after surgery.

MATCHING

1. ____ ambulatory surgery

2. ____ anesthesia

3. ____ anesthesiologist

4. ____ certified registered nurse anesthetist

5. ____ circulating nurse

6. ____ general anesthesia

7. ____ intraoperative phase

8. ____ local anesthesia

9. ____ malignant hyperthermia

10. ____ perioperative

11. ____ perioperative nursing

12. ____ postanesthesia care unit

13. ____ postoperative phase

14. ____ preoperative phase

15. ____ regional anesthesia

16. ____ registered nurse first assistant

17. ____ scrub nurse

a. can be divided into two segments of care: the immediate and the ongoing periods

b. any agent that induces a temporary loss of feeling due to the inhibition of nerve endings in a specific part of the body

c. an area where clients remain until they regain consciousness from the effects of anesthesia; formerly called recovery room

d. a specialized area of practice that describes the provision of care for the surgical client throughout the continuum of care

e. a registered nurse with special qualifications that include knowledge of aseptic technique, instruments and equipment, anatomy and physiology, surgical procedures, and most importantly, promotion of client safety

f. a type of anesthesia in which medication is instilled into or around the nerves to block the transmission of nerve impulses in a particular area or region

g. a medical physician who specializes in anesthesiology

h. same-day or outpatient surgery that can be performed with general or local anesthesia, usually takes less than 2 hours, and requires less than a 3-hour stay in a recovery area

i. a rare autosomal dominant inherited syndrome that causes rigidity of the skeletal muscles and is life threatening

j. begins when the decision for surgical intervention is made and ends when the client is safely transported into the operating room (OR) for the surgical procedure

k. an expanded nursing role requiring additional education, in which the perioperative nurse works as a first assistant during the surgical procedure

l. an advanced practice registered nurse who has been specifically educated in the administration of anesthetic agents

m. begins with the client's entry into the OR and ends when the client is transferred to the recovery room (postanesthesia care unit) or other areas such as the intensive care unit, where immediate postsurgical attention is given

n. the partial or complete loss of sensation with or without a loss of consciousness that results from administration of an anesthetic agent

Copyright © 2004, Elsevier Science (USA). All Rights Reserved.

o. produced by inhalation or by injection of anesthetic drugs into the bloodstream, or a combination of both, and causes the client to lose all sensation and consciousness

p. a registered nurse who assists the client to meet individual needs during all three phases of the surgical experience

q. the term used to describe the preoperative, intraoperative, and postoperative phases of the surgical experience

TRUE OR FALSE

18. ____ Collaborative and independent nursing care prevents complications and promotes optimal outcomes for the surgical client.

19. ____ The scrub nurse coordinates client care, is the client advocate, and manages all activities outside the sterile field.

20. ____ Prior to surgery, the surgeon is required to ask informed consent to have the operative procedure performed.

21. ____ Normal tissue repair and resistance to infection after surgery depend on good nutrition.

22. ____ Clients are less anxious and participate more readily if they know the reasons for perioperative activities.

23. ____ Pain is an unexpected and abnormal response to the surgical procedure.

24. ____ Turning in bed postoperatively improves venous return and respiratory function.

25. ____ In addition to the skin incision, there are many other risk factors that can influence a surgical client's risk for infection.

26. ____ Acetaminophen (Tylenol) is the drug of choice to treat malignant hyperthermia.

27. ____ Urinary retention and urinary tract infections are two common postoperative complications of the urinary system.

FILL-IN-THE-BLANKS

28. A surgery that is performed according to the client's preference with no ill effects occurring due to postponement would be classified as _____ surgery.

29. The _____ phase of anesthesia is begun as soon as the client is brought into the operating room.

30. One advantage of _____ anesthesia is that it can be used for clients of any age and for any surgical procedure.

31. It is the legal responsibility of the _____ to obtain the client's consent before a surgical procedure.

32. Latex allergies have become much more common since the late 1980s with the advent of _____ precautions.

33. Positioning the client for surgery is usually done _____ induction of anesthesia.

34. _____ is a respiratory emergency caused by reflex contractions of pharyngeal muscles, causing spasm of the vocal cords.

35. To encourage maximal lung expansion following surgery, a client should use an _____ _____.

36. A nurse should assess for bladder distention in the postoperative client if the client has not voided for _____ hours.

37. _____ and _____ instructions are given to a client before discharge following surgery.

EXERCISING YOUR CLINICAL JUDGMENT

Mr. Warren, a 61-year-old Afro-Caribbean man, has come to the United States for a second medical opinion after he was diagnosed with prostate cancer. His daughter, who is a nurse, lives in Atlanta.

38. Which of the following nursing diagnoses would you be sure to consider, knowing that Mr. Warren is undergoing surgery for cancer, a potentially incurable problem?
    1. *Anxiety*
    2. *Knowledge deficit*
    3. *Hopelessness*
    4. *Powerlessness*

39. You are providing instructions to Mr. Warren about leg exercises that he can do after surgery to reduce the risk of thrombus formation in his legs. How often should you tell him to perform them?
    1. 1 to 2 times every hour
    2. 5 to 6 times every 1 to 2 hours
    3. 10 to 12 times every 1 to 2 hours
    4. 20 to 25 times every 8 hours

Copyright © 2004, Elsevier Science (USA). All Rights Reserved.

40. Encouraging Mr. Warren to turn, cough, and breathe deep (TCDB) helps him prevent:
    1. being thirsty.
    2. having alveolar collapse and moving secretions to large airway passages for easier expectoration.
    3. having a low heart rate.
    4. having no crackles in his lung fields.

41. You are assisting Mr. Warren to get out of bed for the first time since surgery. Knowing he has an abdominal incision, you would be sure to use which of the following when helping him get up?
    1. Cane to steady himself against
    2. Walker to lean on in case of dizziness
    3. Pillow to use as a splint during movement
    4. Mechanical lift, because he should not stand at all

TEST YOURSELF

42. As part of client preparation just before surgery, you must check the consent form to verify the client has signed it, have the client void, give preoperative medication, and assist the client onto the stretcher to go to the operating room. Which of the following would be best to do first?
    1. Have the client void.
    2. Put the client on the stretcher for needed rest.
    3. Administer the ordered medication.
    4. Verify the client has signed the consent form

43. The preoperative nurse would alert the anesthesiologist or surgeon regarding which of the following health problems that could cause cancellation of a client's elective surgery?
    1. Headache
    2. Sore throat
    3. Heart attack 1 year ago
    4. Chronic lung disease

44. The circulating nurse in the operating room notes that two sponges are missing near the end of a client's surgery. Which of the following actions should the nurse take first?
    1. Call for an x-ray.
    2. Ignore it because the sponges dissolve.
    3. Perform a second count.
    4. Search the floor around the operating table.

45. The nurse would teach the client about which of the following ordered pain medication administration methods that provides for the most continuous relief of pain?
    1. Patient-controlled analgesia
    2. Intermittent nurse-administered IV push medication
    3. Subcutaneous injections
    4. Intramuscular injections

46. A postoperative client with nausea has begun vomiting. The nurse would avoid giving antiemetic medication by which of the following routes?
    1. Intravenous
    2. Intramuscular
    3. Subcutaneous
    4. Oral

Copyright © 2004, Elsevier Science (USA). All Rights Reserved.

ANSWER KEY

CHAPTER 1

1. b
2. d
3. g
4. a
5. c
6. f
7. e
8. T
9. F. Nursing practice is governed by law and standards are set forth by the profession.
10. T
11. T
12. T
13. F. A doctoral program is considered advanced practice education.
14. F. The nurse's role would be critical thinker.
15. T
16. T
17. F. Politics has always permeated both the health care delivery system and the profession of nursing.
18. Middle Ages
19. Florence Nightingale
20. Civil
21. Mary Adelaide Nutting
22. public health
23. primary care, prevention, and community outreach
24. master's degree
25. professional licensure
26. state
27. 1. The Nurse Practice Act forms the legal basis for nursing practice in a specific state. The NLN focuses on the improvement of nursing services and education. The ARN is a specialty nursing organization, and the ANA is the professional organization for nurses.
28. 3. The client advocate role is one in which the nurse protects the rights of clients. In this instance, Kate is protecting the rights of the client whose privacy is being invaded.
29. 2. Many states require that nurses obtain CEUs in order to maintain their professional licensure in that state.
30. 2. A bachelor's degree is the minimum educational degree that must be held in order to become certified by the ANCC as a nurse generalist.
31. 1
32. 3
33. 2
34. 4
35. 4

CHAPTER 2

1. g
2. l
3. q
4. ff
5. w
6. ii
7. aa
8. ee
9. a
10. f
11. m
12. r
13. x
14. bb
15. b
16. t
17. hh
18. u
19. dd
20. c
21. h
22. n
23. z
24. cc
25. jj
26. d
27. s
28. i
29. kk
30. o
31. v
32. e
33. p
34. k
35. v
36. gg
37. ll
38. j
39. T
40. F. It does include refusing to let clients leave the hospital against their wishes.
41. T
42. F. The nurse would be tried under criminal law.
43. T
44. F. An individual state has the power to change the Nurse Practice Act.
45. T
46. T
47. T
48. T
49. F. A terminally ill client should be told of his or her prognosis.
50. F. An ethical dilemma exists when choices are unfavorable.
51. T

Copyright © 2004, Elsevier Science (USA). All Rights Reserved.

52. T
53. battery
54. procedural
55. certification
56. collective bargaining
57. informed consent
58. confidentiality, or privacy
59. incident report
60. ethics
61. culture, life experiences
62. privacy
63. Nonmaleficence
64. medical
65. 4. This is the only option that removes the client from the area and protects the confidentiality of the information being given in report.
66. 1. The CDC is the federal agency responsible for issuing guidelines for infection control.
67. 2. The other options constitute documentation errors.
68. 3
69. 4
70. 2
71. 2
72. 3
73. 4
74. 2
75. 3
76. 3
77. 1
78. 2

CHAPTER 3

1. e
2. i
3. j
4. a
5. f
6. h
7. k
8. c
9. d
10. b
11. g
12. T
13. F. This is an example of stereotyping.
14. T
15. T

16. F. This refers to a person who is past-oriented.
17. T
18. T
19. T
20. T
21. F. Native Americans believe that illness is a price paid for a past or future event.
22. preservation, maintenance
23. accommodation, negotiation
24. Awareness
25. Environmental control
26. Irish
27. African
28. Hispanic
29. Chinese
30. Navajo Indians
31. harmony
32. 3. An adult may choose to continue to closely identify with the group to which his or her parents belonged, or may adopt the ways of the larger culture around him or her.
33. 1. Religion is taken very seriously, and many African-Americans actively participate in church-related activities and believe strongly in the power of prayer.
34. 4
35. 2
36. 3
37. 1
38. 4

CHAPTER 4

1. b
2. g
3. d
4. e
5. f
6. c
7. a
8. i
9. j
10. k
11. l
12. m
13. h
14. n
15. T
16. F. Advanced nurse practitioners include clinical nurse specialists and nurse practitioners. Physician assistants are health care professionals licensed to practice medicine with physician supervision.
17. F. The use of alternative health therapy is growing in typical health care settings.
18. F. Whereas there may be room for debate, many factors influence access and quality of hospital services. Among these factors, consider rural versus urban, system of financing, and types of services offered.
19. T
20. T. Emergency medical services are a means of reducing the response time to emergencies.
21. T. Respite care is designed to relieve the stress and burden of informal caregivers by providing temporary relief of caring for their ill family members.
22. F. The U.S. government's share of the national health care bill was 46%.
23. F. An HMO establishes standards for the quality of care provided.
24. F. Managed care organizations make decisions about what services will be reimbursed, thus rationing health care.
25. T. This is also the age group with the greatest per capita expenditures for health care.
26. T. Hispanics, Asians, and Muslims are among the minority groups whose presence is visibly increasing in the United States.
27. T. As a nurse, you need to understand the economic forces putting pressure on the structure and function of the health care delivery system.
28. F. Cost of care and quality of care are highly interrelated.
29. health behaviors, improved environmental quality
30. Nurses

Copyright © 2004, Elsevier Science (USA). All Rights Reserved.

31. Pharmacists
32. inpatient
33. rural community hospital
34. Rehabilitation
35. Hospice
36. physician's office
37. Adult day care
38. United States
39. preferred provider organization
40. people over 65, disabled people, people with end-stage renal disease
41. Canada
42. Twenty-six
43. American Association of Retired Persons
44. 2. Although none of these sources may provide this service, the goal of a health maintenance organization is most in keeping with this service.
45. 2. Although the managed care organization will make a decision about paying for the medication, a physician must prescribe this medication and will consider his medical history in making the decision.
46. 3. A dietitian is the only one specifically trained to provide dietary counseling.
47. 1. Option 1 is a definition of *rehabilitation*. Options 2, 3, and 4 are incorrect.
48. 3
49. 4
50. 3
51. 4

CHAPTER 5

1. j
2. f
3. h
4. d
5. e
6. a
7. i
8. b
9. c
10. g
11. T
12. T

13. F. It is acceptable when consensus of the nursing profession is that the theory provides an adequate description of reality.
14. F. This is attributed to Leininger.
15. F. The THINK model incorporates five modes of thinking used in combination or simultaneously.
16. T
17. F. Routines are equated with habits. Habits are useful when they free the mind to deal with the more complex aspects of a situation. They are not useful when they substitute for thinking.
18. F. A list of assessment questions is a tool to be used as a reminder and is never intended to be complete.
19. person, nursing
20. theory
21. nurse
22. overuse of the habit mode, anxiety, time, bias, lack of confidence
23. goals, nursing
24. physician's
25. North American Nursing Diagnosis Association
26. 4
27. 3
28. 4
29. 1
30. 1
31. 2
32. 4
33. 1
34. 4
35. 1

CHAPTER 6

1. w
2. z
3. x
4. q
5. u
6. e
7. r
8. v
9. y
10. s

11. t
12. h
13. o
14. f
15. j
16. p
17. n
18. m
19. g
20. i
21. k
22. l
23. d
24. b
25. c
26. a
27. T
28. T
29. F. If the client wishes to maintain privacy or the family is not a reliable source you would not collect data from the family.
30. T
31. T
32. F. The purpose is never only to collect a standard set of data.
33. F. You prepare for termination when you tell the client how much time the interview will take.
34. F. Biographical data may be helpful in accurately anticipating a medical diagnosis.
35. F. The medical history helps the nurse anticipate nursing needs.
36. T
37. T
38. F. Exercise tolerance is related to the respiratory and cardiovascular systems as well.
39. F. However, subjective data are documented in an objective manner, without including your opinions.
40. T
41. restoration
42. potential for, potential rate of, evidence of
43. location, quality, chronology, setting, severity, aggravating or alleviating factors, associated factors

Copyright © 2004, Elsevier Science (USA). All Rights Reserved.

44. Rapport
45. chronology
46. nutritional-metabolic
47. activity-exercise
48. self-perception/self-concept
49. 4
50. 2
51. 2
52. 3
53. 1
54. 2
55. 2
56. 2
57. 3
58. 3

CHAPTER 7

1. d
2. h
3. e
4. i
5. j
6. k
7. g
8. l
9. m
10. n
11. a
12. f
13. o
14. p
15. c
16. b
17. F. Vital signs must be evaluated and compared with the client's baseline.
18. T
19. T
20. T
21. F. The oral thermometer must be placed in the pocket created by the frenulum under the tongue.
22. F. Clean from clean to dirty; that is, from the end to the bulb.
23. F. A heart rate of 100 with exercise or anxiety that returns to normal with rest is normal.
24. T
25. T
26. F. Head injuries can cause bradycardia.
27. F. The blood volume is also a factor.

28. F. The carotid is not routinely used to count the pulse. Massage of the carotid can cause a reflex slowing of the heart rate.
29. T
30. T
31. T
32. Vital signs
33. thermoregulation
34. glass
35. tympanic
36. metabolic rate
37. increase
38. pulsus paradoxus
39. resistance
40. contraction
41. relaxation
42. two thirds
43. 2
44. 1
45. 2
46. 1
47. 3
48. 3
49. 3
50. 1
51. 2
52. 3
53. 2
54. 2
55. 4
56. 1
57. 2
58. 4
59. 1
60. 2
61. 1
62. 3
63. 3

CHAPTER 8

1. e
2. f
3. d
4. n
5. g
6. h
7. i
8. j
9. c
10. b
11. a
12. k
13. l

14. m
15. F. A good quality stethoscope has a thick wall.
16. F. A stethoscope does not amplify, it simply blocks out other sounds.
17. F. You can begin the physical exam in any position.
18. T
19. F. The heart is on the left side.
20. T
21. F. This information is a form of orientation to time, but can only be evaluated in the context of the information.
22. T
23. T
24. F. PERRLA tells you more about motor function than the ability to see clearly.
25. T
26. F. Angle the ophthalmoscope toward the nose.
27. F. The thyroid should be soft.
28. T
29. T
30. T
31. T
32. T
33. F. An apical radial pulse deficit usually occurs with irregular cardiac rhythms.
34. T
35. F. A grade 6 is the loudest murmur.
36. F. A bruit is never normal.
37. T
38. F. Identifying hypoactive bowel sounds is a subjective judgment dependent on your ability to recognize normal sounds.
39. T
40. T
41. light palpation
42. percussion
43. auscultation
44. cognitive function
45. natural
46. Crepitus
47. 2, 30, 60
48. Rinne
49. gingivitis
50. Kussmaul
51. discontinuous
52. Deep tendon

Copyright © 2004, Elsevier Science (USA). All Rights Reserved.

53. Papanicolaou smear
54. prostate
55. varicocele
56. 1, 6, 10, and 11 are essential.
   1. Essential. Assessing for adventitious sounds will help you know the seriousness of her condition, anticipate complications, and monitor progress.
   2. Nonessential. However, you will probably want to gather some information about her mental status such as orientation to person, place, and time. Gather enough information that you can recognize if her condition changes.
   3. Nonessential. Assess the radial and pedal pulses. Assess the radial pulse to evaluate the rate and rhythm of the heart. If the rhythm is irregular, assess the apical pulse. Assess the pedal pulses to evaluate the circulation in the feet. It would not be surprising for a 90-year-old to have diminished circulation in the feet.
   4. Nonessential. However, you do want to listen for bowel sounds and assess for abdominal distention. The stress of illness can slow the bowels and cause distention.
   5. Nonessential. The rectal examination is never routine for a general duty nurse.
   6. Essential. Skin assessment in the elderly is important especially when the person will be confined to bed.
   7. Nonessential. However, you will want to note some information about range of motion and the ability to move about safely in the environment.
   8. Nonessential. However, most nurses will usually note the condition of the toenails in the elderly. Health teaching needs can be met and sometimes a podiatrist referral can be made.
   9. Nonessential. However, you do want to gather some information about the client's functional level of vision and hearing and the use of glasses or hearing aids.
   10. Essential. Cardiac and respiratory problems are closely interrelated and should always be assessed together.
   11. Essential. Anytime you listen to the heart one of the things you are listening for is murmurs. The presence of most murmurs will not appreciably change your nursing care.

57. 4
58. 2
59. 3
60. 1
61. 3
62. 1
63. 3
64. 2
65. 2
66. 4
67. 4
68. 2
69. 3
70. 3
71. 3
72. 2
73. 3
74. 2
75. 2
76. 1
77. 2
78. 3
79. 2
80. 2

CHAPTER 9

1. g
2. j
3. h
4. i
5. n
6. b

7. d
8. m
9. l
10. e
11. c
12. f
13. a
14. k
15. T
16. T
17. F. NANDA
18. T
19. F. The nine patterns of response are exchanging, communicating, relating, valuing, choosing, moving, perceiving, knowing, and feeling.
20. T
21. T
22. F. qualifier
23. T
24. F. Nursing diagnoses should be discussed with the client.
25. second
26. Omaha
27. diagnostic label
28. wellness
29. clusters
30. differentiating
31. defining characteristic
32. libel
33. overdiagnosing
34. 1. This is an actual nursing diagnosis, not "risk for," and lists specific related factors.
35. 2. The client cannot retain urine with a catheter in place.
36. 2. This would be a "risk for" diagnosis. The "related to" factors must relate to the client's situation.
37. 4. The diagnosis would be written as *Risk for infection.*
38. 4
39. 1
40. 2
41. 1
42. 3

CHAPTER 10

1. b
2. m
3. l
4. e
5. k
6. a

7. f
8. p
9. n
10. h
11. j
12. c
13. o
14. d
15. i
16. g
17. F. Planning is ongoing throughout the client health care experience.
18. F. Each care plan is individualized.
19. F. Whereas other disciplines may in some cases assume primary responsibility for some aspects of the client's care, the nurse has a role in the provision of that care.
20. T
21. F. Physical needs may be secondary to other needs at different stages of the client's experience.
22. T
23. T
24. T
25. T
26. F. Outcomes or nursing diagnoses may also be revised.
27. F. The client and family must be asked.
28. T
29. T
30. T
31. changes
32. physiological integrity
33. nursing, multidisciplinary
34. accountable
35. sensitive
36. Likert, five
37. communication
38. partially
39. resolved
40. barrier
41. indicators
42. 2
43. 4
44. 2
45. 4
46. 4
47. 3
48. 4
49. 1

50. 2
51. 3
52. 2
53. 2

CHAPTER 11

1. d
2. f
3. k
4. p
5. o
6. a
7. i
8. j
9. b
10. l
11. c
12. g
13. h
14. n
15. e
16. m
17. T
18. F. Errors are documented in the client's chart.
19. F. Abbreviations vary from geographical area or specialty.
20. F. Charting should be as brief as possible, stripped to essential components.
21. T
22. T
23. T
24. documentation, communication
25. standards
26. Black
27. client's
28. client
29. orientation
30. observations
31. 1. Narrative charting is a method of charting that provides information in the form of statements that describe events surrounding client care.
32. 2. Recording of information should be sequential.
33. 3. A discharge note is done when client is released from the hospital.
34. 3
35. 4

36. 4
37. 2
38. 1

CHAPTER 12

1. c
2. s
3. p
4. m
5. h
6. g
7. r
8. d
9. i
10. k
11. e
12. l
13. n
14. o
15. f
16. b
17. a
18. q
19. j
20. T
21. F. This is Travelbee's theory.
22. T
23. F. A person's personal space is culturally determined.
24. T
25. T
26. F. You should ask the client to consider what might be the best thing to do.
27. T
28. ethical, professional
29. Positive
30. body language
31. presenting reality
32. talking
33. silence
34. Active
35. 1. The nurse asks "why" of the client, thereby asking for a reason for feelings and behaviors when the client may not know the reason.
36. 3. The nurse lets the client know that what was said was unclear.
37. 1. The nurse invites the client to select a topic.
38. 1
39. 1

Copyright © 2004, Elsevier Science (USA). All Rights Reserved.

40. 4
41. 1
42. 4

CHAPTER 13

1. g
2. d
3. a
4. h
5. f
6. c
7. e
8. b
9. T
10. T
11. F. Clients may only be able to comprehend the steps of a carefully prescribed routine.
12. F. Literacy is an important consideration when using written instructions.
13. T
14. T
15. F. Written supplemental materials reinforce learning.
16. F. Some clients prefer not to know.
17. F. Other nursing diagnoses can also apply.
18. T
19. T
20. individual
21. group
22. printed
23. reinforce learning
24. active participant
25. short-term
26. long-term
27. 3. Adult learning is purposeful.
28. 3. For adults, learning must have a purpose.
29. 1. Motivation is greatest in clients who recognize their learning needs and perceive the available teaching as meaningful.
30. 2
31. 1
32. 1
33. 1
34. 2
35. 2

36. 1
37. 1
38. 3

CHAPTER 14

1. b
2. e
3. l
4. f
5. g
6. h
7. c
8. k
9. i
10. a
11. d
12. j
13. T
14. T
15. F. A mission statement is written.
16. T
17. T
18. T
19. T
20. F. policy
21. concurrent
22. improved
23. health
24. leaders
25. organization
26. organizational chart
27. quality
28. outcomes
29. Policies, procedures
30. cost
31. 1. The nurse–manager can delegate this task to the charge nurse, who is responsible for the daily operation of the unit. Although the nurse–manager role involves managing personnel, this usually involves evaluation of performance and possibly hiring and firing personnel. The other options do not address the immediate problem in an effective manner.
32. 2. Because the change enhanced the level of service rendered to the client, this is an example of an improvement in quality.

33. 3. Projected revenue is the anticipated income after considering the cost of both staffing and supplies. The ability to anticipate future needs is referred to as forecasting. Concepts of negotiation and lobbying do not apply to the situation described.
34. 2
35. 3
36. 4
37. 3
38. 1
39. 4
40. 3

CHAPTER 15

1. a
2. h
3. b
4. g
5. c
6. d
7. e
8. m
9. l
10. f
11. i
12. o
13. j
14. n
15. k
16. p
17. r
18. q
19. s
20. T
21. T
22. T
23. F. Ethical guidelines should still be followed.
24. T
25. F. There is a relationship, but not necessarily causation.
26. F. The abstract is a short summary only.
27. T
28. T
29. T
30. F. It can.
31. T
32. F. Valuable information can still be obtained.

Copyright © 2004, Elsevier Science (USA). All Rights Reserved.

33. T
34. T
35. T
36. Nursing research
37. Florence Nightingale
38. human subjects
39. case study
40. variables
41. random
42. reduction
43. extraneous
44. maturation
45. Transferability
46. 1
47. 4
48. 2
49. 1
50. 4
51. 1
52. 1
53. 2

CHAPTER 16

1. o
2. m
3. h
4. q
5. b
6. k
7. e
8. c
9. d
10. p
11. a
12. f
13. l
14. g
15. i
16. n
17. r
18. j
19. T
20. T
21. F. Tasks can derive from cultural patterns as well.
22. T
23. T
24. T
25. F. The preschool child gains weight more slowly.
26. T
27. F. Children of this age group have many fears.
28. T
29. T

30. F. Boys are affected more than girls.
31. F. Most cases of short stature result from heredity.
32. T
33. T
34. head, heel
35. 4
36. separation anxiety
37. 12
38. Phenylketonuria
39. ectomorphic, endomorphic
40. preschool-aged
41. head, collisions
42. 5
43. identity, identity diffusion
44. health care
45. psychosocial
46. comply or adhere
47. 4. The other toys are best used with children younger than 12 months of age.
48. 2. The other strategies should be avoided.
49. 3. The client cannot read (age 33 months) and has a language barrier.
50. 3. A nap should be planned around lunchtime.
51. 3
52. 3
53. 1
54. 2
55. 3
56. 4
57. 3
58. 3
59. 1
60. 2
61. 1
62. 3
63. 2
64. 4
65. 3

CHAPTER 17

1. b
2. g
3. e
4. f
5. d
6. h
7. c
8. a
9. T

10. T
11. F. The young adult stage is intimacy versus isolation.
12. T
13. F. It is usually difficult to detect.
14. F. One in every five deaths is related to cigarette smoking.
15. T
16. T. This is especially true for clients in high-risk groups
17. T
18. generativity, stagnation
19. seasons
20. infectious diseases
21. Ageism
22. depressed
23. Poverty
24. unintentional, homicide
25. individualized
26. incontinence
27. 4 .The individual must balance the feeling that life is personally satisfying and socially meaningful with the feeling that life is without meaning.
28. 3. Midlife crisis is a stressful life period during middle adulthood, precipitated by the review and reevaluation of one's past, including goals, during which the person experiences inner turmoil and self-doubt.
29. 3. To persuade clients to change their behaviors, it is first necessary to identify their beliefs relevant to the high-risk behavior and to provide information based on this foundation.
30. 4
31. 3
32. 2
33. 1
34. 1
35. 3

CHAPTER 18

1. g
2. j
3. i
4. k
5. a

Copyright © 2004, Elsevier Science (USA). All Rights Reserved.

6. d
7. c
8. b
9. n
10. f
11. o
12. m
13. h
14. l
15. q
16. e
17. p
18. T
19. T
20. F. Health is a fundamental right of all people.
21. F. Not all diseases can be cured.
22. T
23. F. Population health addresses the five determinants of health: biology, behaviors, physical environment, social environment, and public policies and interventions.
24. T
25. T
26. World Health Organization
27. quality, years
28. choice, passively
29. diagnosis
30. health-illness continuum
31. population
32. perception
33. medical
34. 1
35. 1
36. 2
37. 4
38. 2
39. 1

CHAPTER 19

1. d
2. f
3. o
4. i
5. m
6. k
7. h
8. c
9. p
10. e
11. a
12. b
13. q

14. l
15. g
16. j
17. n
18. T
19. T
20. F. They do interfere.
21. T
22. F. They may conflict with interventions.
23. T
24. T
25. T
26. F. Client and family should also be involved.
27. T
28. reasoned action
29. risk factors
30. lifestyle, family
31. medical
32. knowledge
33. Values clarification
34. reinforcing, motivating
35. denial
36. Discharge
37. social
38. 1. In this stage, the person does not intend to change a high-risk behavior in the foreseeable future.
39. 2. He disliked having to go to the bathroom so frequently because of medication effects.
40. 3. An educational plan must be focused on increasing awareness of the relationships between the client's specific unhealthy lifestyles and the development of health problems.
41. 4. The single most influential factor in increasing participation in effective management of a therapeutic regimen is the relationship with the health care provider.
42. 1
43. 3
44. 2
45. 4
46. 3

CHAPTER 20

1. d
2. z

3. p
4. a
5. y
6. o
7. l
8. b
9. k
10. u
11. m
12. e
13. q
14. t
15. x
16. g
17. v
18. n
19. c
20. i
21. j
22. f
23. r
24. s
25. h
26. w
27. T
28. T
29. F. The drugs reach the liver first, called the first-pass effect.
30. T
31. F. It varies according to facility policy.
32. T
33. T
34. F. Sufficient body fluid is needed to transport drugs and their metabolites.
35. T
36. Drug Enforcement
37. Drug tolerance
38. Enteric-coated
39. X
40. body weight
41. *constipation, diarrhea*
42. superinfection
43. 30
44. 3. The client should develop and use a reminder system, if needed, because omitted doses can jeopardize health. The statements in the other options are false.
45. 2. Standing or sitting up slowly allows the blood vessels time to adjust in caliber to the position change

Copyright © 2004, Elsevier Science (USA). All Rights Reserved.

and may help decrease adverse symptoms. Options 1 and 3 will make dizziness worse. The client should take the medication at bedtime if dizziness is a chronic problem.
46. 4. The term *sublingual* means "under the tongue," making it the only correct response.
47. 1. Adverse medication effects are more likely to occur with increasing age because the body may not metabolize and excrete them as easily.
48. 1
49. 3
50. 2
51. 4
52. 2

CHAPTER 21

1. i
2. h
3. e
4. a
5. k
6. n
7. p
8. q
9. b
10. m
11. o
12. d
13. j
14. l
15. g
16. c
17. s
18. r
19. f
20. T
21. T
22. F. Measles is an airborne infection.
23. T
24. T
25. F. It is a left shift.
26. T
27. F. Anxiety can reduce protection.
28. T
29. T
30. convalescence
31. reservoir
32. Opportunistic
33. environmental
34. localized
35. dirty
36. hand hygiene
37. steam
38. feces
39. Droplet
40. 1. The others are localized signs of infection.
41. 3. The environment has other children, and hand-washing is a fundamental procedure to reduce transmission of organisms.
42. 2. Viruses, such as influenza, require droplet precautions.
43. 4. The sites should be recultured or new sites of infection should be looked for.
44. 1
45. 1
46. 4
47. 2
48. 3

CHAPTER 22

1. f
2. e
3. a
4. h
5. i
6. g
7. d
8. b
9. c
10. T
11. T
12. F. Cigarette smoking is the leading cause of fatal residential fires.
13. T
14. F. Most back injuries develop slowly over time.
15. T
16. T
17. T
18. F. The child's age is also a consideration when buying a car seat.
19. T
20. falls
21. aspiration
22. Poisons
23. accidental
24. occupational
25. money
26. infants, toddlers
27. prevention
28. grounded
29. rescue, alarm, confine, extinguish
30. 2. Measures to promote home safety may include using nonskid rugs or tacking down throw rugs to prevent slips and falls.
31. 2. Safety practices to prevent burns, such as positioning pans with handles toward the back of the stove while cooking, should be in place.
32. 4. A person's cognitive and perceptual abilities are crucial to promoting safety.
33. 3. Multipurpose extinguisher are for type A, B, and C fires.
34. 3
35. 4
36. 2

CHAPTER 23

1. i
2. a
3. d
4. b
5. s
6. q
7. c
8. m
9. n
10. g
11. e
12. r
13. f
14. o
15. h
16. j
17. p
18. l
19. k
20. T
21. F. Most digestion and absorption occur in the small intestine.
22. T

Copyright © 2004, Elsevier Science (USA). All Rights Reserved.

23. F. A high-fiber diet contains cereals and raw fruits and vegetables.
24. F. Positive nitrogen balance and anabolism occur when the body is storing protein.
25. T
26. T
27. F. The RDA is meant to meet the needs of healthy individuals.
28. T
29. T
30. T
31. Digestion
32. fiber
33. 4
34. Vitamins
35. minerals
36. diet history
37. Food Guide Pyramid
38. protein
39. Nutrition Facts food label
40. fruits, vegetables
41. Polyphenols
42. 3. The client has well-fitting dentures and no evidence of neuromuscular disease.
43. 2. Physical factors that can interfere with nutrition include circumstances that interfere with the ability to shop, cook, and eat. Arthritis could limit the ability to do all of these.
44. 1. The family should be assessed first as a possible resource for shopping and/or food preparation. Option 2 could be costly, whereas option 3 may not be necessary at this time. Option 4 does not solve possible difficulty in shopping when the client has arthritis.
45. 4. The Food Guide Pyramid uses a graphic design that is useful in teaching clients about the types and amounts of foods to include in the daily diet. It is easy to understand and follow.
46. 1
47. 2
48. 4
49. 3
50. 2
51. 1

CHAPTER 24

1. d
2. e
3. a
4. f
5. g
6. b
7. c
8. T
9. F. Ketones are positive and nitrogen balance is negative.
10. T
11. F. It occurs over months or years.
12. T
13. T
14. T
15. F. At least 2 pounds per month is considered successful.
16. T
17. F. They should be avoided.
18. medulla
19. B_{12}
20. iron
21. 34
22. 10
23. pharyngeal
24. 170
25. clear
26. 2
27. limited or restricted
28. 3. Zinc is the element that has an effect of increasing the ability to taste. The other minerals listed do not have this property.
29. 1. Clients with cancer and AIDS tend to eat better in the morning.
30. 2. These foods can cause further irritation.
31. 4. Both hemoglobin and hematocrit will reflect increased iron intake.
32. 1
33. 3
34. 2
35. 4
36. 2

CHAPTER 25

1. a
2. u
3. f

4. c
5. e
6. b
7. h
8. g
9. j
10. q
11. t
12. s
13. o
14. n
15. r
16. p
17. k
18. m
19. i
20. d
21. l
22. T
23. T
24. T
25. F. Hypokalemia is a result of high volume urine output.
26. T
27. T
28. F. It cannot be measured.
29. T
30. T
31. F. It's given primarily for fluid replacement.
32. F. Sodium is present in this solution (0.45%).
33. T
34. T
35. T
36. retention
37. water-soluble
38. decompression, obstruction
39. third spacing
40. high Fowler's
41. Normal saline
42. distal
43. 18
44. at the site, away from
45. blood return
46. 3. Others represent deficient fluid volume.
47. 1. Sodium would be low; others show normal or high values.
48. 1. Crackles are consistent with overload.
49. 2. 20 times 60 divided by 60 = 20.
50. 3. Weight is reliable indicator of fluid status.

Copyright © 2004, Elsevier Science (USA). All Rights Reserved.

51. 4
52. 3
53. 3
54. 1
55. 1
56. 2
57. 2
58. 2
59. 3
60. 2

CHAPTER 26

1. f
2. k
3. i
4. l
5. b
6. j
7. c
8. h
9. d
10. g
11. m
12. n
13. e
14. o
15. a
16. F. They may or may not be related.
17. F. Yellow indicates that a wound is not ready to heal.
18. T
19. T
20. F. Wounds cannot heal when infected.
21. F. Yellow drainage does not always means the wound is infected.
22. T
23. Protection
24. red, yellow, black
25. pressure ulcer
26. perioperative, postoperative
27. clock
28. sutures, staples
29. enterostomal
30. 2. A Stage II ulcer may look like a blister or shallow crater.
31. 2. The erythrocyte sedimentation rate can help assess the client's inflammation, infectious, or necrotic processes.

32. 4. *Impaired skin integrity:* It is a state in which an individual has altered body tissue.
33. 3
34. 1
35. 4
36. 2
37. 1

CHAPTER 27

1. f
2. h
3. c
4. a
5. g
6. d
7. e
8. b
9. F. Fever may also be caused by inflammation without infection.
10. T
11. T
12. T
13. F. Hypothermic clients exhibit a high alcohol or other drug intake
14. T
15. T
16. T
17. F. Besides identifying bacteria in the blood (bacteremia), blood cultures can identify viruses in the blood (viremia).
18. F. Blood cultures are drawn through a central line IV site only if the central line is suspected to be the source of the infection.
19. T
20. F. Convulsions in infants are associated with a temperature of 102° to 104° F or higher.
21. T
22. T
23. F. Hypothermia is the result.
24. T
25. T
26. effervescence, plateau, defervescence
27. 10%
28. increased
29. dry skin, hypotension, tachycardia, vomiting, diarrhea.

30. warmth, shivering, vasodilation
31. Chronic fever
32. tinnitus, bruising
33. liver
34. conduction
35. convection
36. hyperthermia
37. Defervescence
38. hypothalamus
39. antipyretics, physical cooling
40. abdominal distention, bowel sounds, nausea
41. 1. If the client has an elevated temperature, monitoring every 4 hours is usually sufficient.
42. 1. Fever is a host defense response that frequently occurs in hospitalized people either from the primary diagnosis or from complications.
43. 2
44. 2
45. 3
46. 1

CHAPTER 28

1. f
2. h
3. g
4. i
5. r
6. o
7. b
8. e
9. c
10. n
11. q
12. p
13. d
14. l
15. m
16. a
17. j
18. k
19. T
20. T
21. F. It can be done with a consistent bowel training program.
22. T

Copyright © 2004, Elsevier Science (USA). All Rights Reserved.

23. F. Exercise can prevent constipation.
24. T
25. F. Motor sensory disturbances can lead to constipation and fecal incontinence.
26. T
27. T
28. F. Mental depression can contribute by slowing bodily processes.
29. fiber
30. loosen
31. Diverticulosis
32. mastication
33. fat, fiber
34. liquid
35. 40
36. flatulence
37. person or individual
38. dependence
39. 3
40. 4
41. 2
42. 1
43. 1
44. 3
45. 2
46. 2
47. 4

CHAPTER 29

1. m
2. u
3. k
4. l
5. a
6. h
7. t
8. v
9. b
10. r
11. s
12. e
13. n
14. g
15. d
16. i
17. p
18. q
19. w
20. c
21. f
22. o
23. j

24. F. The bladder is under voluntary control of the sympathetic nervous system.
25. T
26. T
27. F. Urinary incontinence is not normal.
28. T
29. F. It is under control of the sympathetic nervous system.
30. T
31. T
32. T
33. F. Small amounts of blood are not visible.
34. F. A minimum of 10 cc is needed.
35. F. Antibiotics are not always indicated.
36. vesicoureteral
37. detrusor
38. urea, creatinine, uric acid, bilirubin, metabolites of hormones
39. sodium, potassium
40. peristalsis
41. inflammation, infection, obstruction
42. frequency
43. 150, 500
44. Voiding urogram
45. Creatinine
46. Stress
47. functional, total
48. prompted voiding
49. habit training
50. Kegel exercises
51. 1. Indwelling urinary catheters are a major cause of urinary tract infection in hospitalized clients. For this reason, it is important to remove the catheter as soon as possible after surgery.
52. 2. Taking a deep breath relaxes the abdominal muscles, which may make catheter removal easier. Each of the other options represents an activity in which the client could bear down, which could increase discomfort.
53. 3. Clients are expected to void no later than 8 hours after catheter removal. It is very important to calculate the

appropriate time for each client
54. 4. Increasing fluid intake will increase the volume of blood filtered in the kidneys, resulting in increased urine output. The larger volume of urine often makes it easier to void following catheter removal.
55. 2
56. 1
57. 4
58. 1
59. 4
60. 4
61. 2
62. 3
63. 2
64. 1

CHAPTER 30

1. f
2. b
3. a
4. e
5. c
6. g
7. h
8. d
9. F. The melanocyte, which is located at the base of the epidermis, produces melanin, one of the pigments responsible for skin color.
10. T
11. F. Thick, yellow nails could indicate fungal infection.
12. F. It would reinforce a client's dependence.
13. T
14. T
15. T
16. T
17. Self-care
18. vitamin D
19. systemic
20. caries
21. blood
22. carcinomas
23. bed bath
24. wide-toothed, pick
25. 2. *Bathing/hygiene self-care deficit:* Impaired ability to perform or complete

Copyright © 2004, Elsevier Science (USA). All Rights Reserved.

bathing/hygiene activities for
oneself
26. 2. A hot-water bath helps
relieve muscle spasm and
muscle tension.
27. 4. *Disturbed thought processes*
related to loss of memory
28. 2
29. 1
30. 2
31. 1
32. 4

CHAPTER 31

1. j
2. h
3. g
4. l
5. m
6. i
7. o
8. f
9. c
10. b
11. e
12. d
13. n
14. k
15. a
16. T
17. F. Vertebral bone decreases in
postmenopausal women.
18. T
19. T
20. F. A slight limitation of ROM
is acceptable.
21. T
22. T
23. osteoclastic
24. atrophy
25. metatarsus varus
26. muscle weakness
27. Crepitus
28. Physical
29. Rehabilitation
30. 1. *Impaired physical mobility*
related to healing hip fracture
31. 2. The physical therapist
focuses on increasing mobility
skills.
32. 1. ROM exercises are isotonic
exercises.
33. 1
34. 3
35. 1

36. 3
37. 3

CHAPTER 32

1. c
2. b
3. d
4. o
5. r
6. k
7. e
8. j
9. p
10. a
11. h
12. l
13. m
14. f
15. g
16. n
17. q
18. i
19. s
20. T
21. T
22. F. The longer the person is
immobile, the higher the risk
of complications of disuse.
23. F. Local circulation is impaired.
24. F. Orthostatic intolerance is a
drop in systolic blood
pressure.
25. T
26. T
27. Disuse
28. longer
29. energy
30. ulcers
31. orthostatic hypotension
32. calculi
33. 1, 2, hours
34. 1. In a friction injury, the
epidermal layer of the skin is
rubbed off.
35. 2. For moderate *Risk for disuse
syndrome,* assess and
intervene every 2 to 4 hours.
36. 3. *Risk for disuse syndrome:* A
state in which an individual is
at risk for deterioration of
body systems as the result of
prescribed or unavoidable
musculoskeletal inactivity.
37. 4
38. 2

39. 1
40. 2
41. 1

CHAPTER 33

1. b
2. c
3. i
4. d
5. a
6. h
7. j
8. f
9. e
10. g
11. k
12. r
13. o
14. v
15. q
16. m
17. l
18. n
19. u
20. p
21. s
22. t
23. T
24. T
25. F. Tidal volume is the amount
of air moved with normal flow
of air in and out of the lungs.
26. T
27. F. Sitting or standing straight
without support is the
optimum position.
28. T
29. F. Nicotine patches, along with
counseling and support, have a
30% success rate.
30. F. The pain of fractured ribs
restricts the chest wall
movement.
31. T
32. T
33. F. In a stable client in a home
environment, clean technique
is appropriate.
34. F. Oxygen saturation should be
95% or greater.
35. diaphragm
36. Elastic recoil
37. Surfactant
38. Sighing
39. Dead space

Copyright © 2004, Elsevier Science (USA). All Rights Reserved.

40. glottis
41. complete blood count
42. forced vital capacity
43. 95
44. Obtundation
45. Thick, tenacious
46. Altered breathing pattern
47. deoxygenated hemoglobin
48. Naloxone (Narcan)
49. 2. Because this is a low-flow oxygen system, the client needs to breathe additional air in order to inhale sufficient air to meet the needs of the lungs. The other responses are incorrect rationales for this question.
50. 1. With hypoventilation, the lungs do not expand as fully as necessary, and because of this, the respiratory rate increases in an attempt to compensate.
51. 3. The inhaler should be activated at the same time as the client takes a deep breath so that the medication is dispersed well into the respiratory tree and does not accumulate in the mouth and upper airway.
52. 2
53. 3
54. 1
55. 1
56. 4
57. 4
58. 1
59. 1
60. 4
61. 1
62. 2
63. 2

CHAPTER 34

1. f
2. g
3. p
4. a
5. r
6. i
7. b
8. j
9. l
10. m
11. o

12. d
13. n
14. h
15. q
16. e
17. c
18. k
19. T
20. F. Greater stroke volume is produced.
21. T
22. F. Decreased blood flow to tissues and decreased oxygen-carrying capacity of hemoglobin results.
23. T
24. T
25. F. They cause inflammation and scarring of cardiac tissue.
26. T
27. T
28. T
29. 5, 6
30. Cocaine, amphetamines
31. atherosclerosis
32. 140/90
33. cerebrovascular accident
34. left
35. Iron
36. aspirin
37. vasoconstriction
38. diet, exercise, smoking
39. 1. Rest periods should be interspersed with activities.
40. 3. Sauces often contain salt.
41. 4. This will help to prevent orthostatic hypotension, a risk of this type of medication.
42. 2. Any activity that tenses abdominal or chest muscles can cause the Valsalva maneuver.
43. 1
44. 4
45. 3
46. 4
47. 1

CHAPTER 35

1. k
2. a
3. m
4. v
5. s
6. c

7. h
8. q
9. t
10. p
11. e
12. r
13. f
14. x
15. i
16. w
17. u
18. g
19. b
20. n
21. d
22. j
23. l
24. o
25. y
26. T
27. F. A depressed client may stay in bed an adequate number of hours but may feel mentally drained.
28. T
29. T
30. F. It is intrinsic.
31. F. The person will return to a restful state if left alone.
32. T
33. T
34. zeitgeber
35. Melatonin
36. caffeine
37. REM
38. 2
39. Narcolepsy
40. back
41. valerian
42. 1. Because it has such a long half-life, caffeine taken late in the day may increase insomnia and nighttime arousals.
43. 4. Because the half-life of nicotine is 1 to 2 hours, the person who smokes more than one cigarette within an hour of bedtime may delay sleep onset.
44. 2. The client should go to bed only when sleepy, refrain from daytime naps, and set the alarm for the same time each day.

Copyright © 2004, Elsevier Science (USA). All Rights Reserved.

45. 4. They are practiced for 20 minutes, can be used during the night as well, and may be enhanced with deep breathing exercises.
46. 2
47. 1
48. 4
49. 3
50. 2

CHAPTER 36

1. s
2. dd
3. l
4. hh
5. m
6. u
7. y
8. t
9. ff
10. w
11. aa
12. bb
13. ii
14. v
15. n
16. h
17. d
18. b
19. c
20. ee
21. k
22. j
23. cc
24. i
25. a
26. r
27. x
28. p
29. q
30. g
31. z
32. e
33. gg
34. o
35. f
36. T
37. F. This refers to somatic pain.
38. T
39. T
40. T
41. F. Pain is the same in the elderly as for any other population.

42. T
43. diagnostic, response
44. Referred
45. learned
46. Chronic
47. pain rating scale
48. neuropathic
49. neuropathic
50. 3. Cultural expectations can mold the meaning of pain and the subsequent behaviors; your lack of understanding of those expectations can interfere with an accurate pain assessment.
51. 4. The correct nursing diagnosis is *Chronic pain* related to malignant disease. progression
52. 4. Rescue dosing involves giving as-needed doses of an immediate-release analgesic in response to the breakthrough pain in addition to the scheduled analgesic dosage.
53. 2
54. 2
55. 4
56. 3
57. 2

CHAPTER 37

1. i
2. j
3. m
4. l
5. c
6. b
7. g
8. f
9. e
10. a
11. n
12. d
13. k
14. h
15. F. Sensory deficits occur most commonly in older adults.
16. T
17. T
18. T
19. F. They are tests to determine conduction or sensorineural hearing loss.

20. T
21. F. A hearing aid may be damaged from radiation.
22. somesthetic
23. Strabismus
24. conductive
25. age
26. Snellen
27. staining
28. overload
29. 1. Night blindness is one of the most distressing symptoms of cataracts because it interferes with night driving and seeing in darkened rooms.
30. 3. *Disturbed sensory perception: visual* (cataract causing visual problems for her)
31. 2. *Risk for injury:* teaching client how to care for eye to prevent it from becoming injured
32. 3
33. 1
34. 2
35. 2
36. 1

CHAPTER 38

1. i
2. d
3. k
4. g
5. l
6. a
7. h
8. j
9. b
10. e
11. f
12. c
13. T
14. F. Nonverbal communication, such as eye contact, facial expression, and head movements, may have different meanings in different cultures.
15. T
16. T Important aspect
17. T
18. T
19. T

Copyright © 2004, Elsevier Science (USA). All Rights Reserved.

20. F. Psychiatric illness can affect communication with others.
21. T
22. F. A risk is that both think they understand each other when in fact they do not.
23. neurological
24. Telegraphic
25. global
26. dysphonia
27. tracheostomy
28. Broca's
29. esophageal
30. receptive
31. Powerlessness
32. physical
33. 1. If there is incongruity between behavior and the spoken word, it requires further assessment.
34. 3. When using an interpreter, always direct your questions and attention to the client, not the interpreter.
35. 4. The client may not understand explanations of procedures and treatment, and it raises an ethical concern if the client cannot fully understand a consent form or completely understand the teaching related to an informed consent solicited before a test, procedure, or surgery.
36. 2. Expected outcome appropriate for diagnosis of *Impaired communication* in this situation is that he expresses satisfaction with the communication process.
37. 1
38. 1
39. 3
40. 4
41. 1

CHAPTER 39

1. e
2. g
3. n
4. f

5. l
6. j
7. i
8. a
9. o
10. c
11. k
12. m
13. p
14. b
15. d
16. h
17. q
18. F. Confusion can occur in younger people, although incidence increases with age.
19. T
20. T
21. F. The client may not be able to judge safety issues with any degree of insight.
22. T
23. T
24. T
25. F. Attention span is included in the assessment.
26. T
27. F. Bright colors or symbols should be used to identify room and/or bathroom for a client with chronic confusion.
28. frontal, temporal
29. acute
30. night
31. circadian
32. Alzheimer's
33. abstract
34. apraxia
35. fever
36. remote
37. injury
38. 2. The other options could increase the risk of injury.
39. 3. The other options could increase anxiety, which could worsen confusion.
40. 1. The other options could impair the client's ability to get restful sleep.
41. 4. Appropriate lighting and visible reminders are most helpful.
42. 4
43. 2
44. 3

45. 1
46. 2

CHAPTER 40

1. e
2. c
3. f
4. b
5. a
6. d
7. T
8. T
9. T
10. T
11. F. This demonstrates a positive correlation.
12. T
13. F. Socioeconomic status has a direct relationship to self-concept.
14. T
15. T
16. F. This is done only when indicated, such as with health problems that typically affect self-concept.
17. body image
18. self-actualization
19. identity
20. power, control
21. emotional, cognitive, perceptual
22. parenting
23. self-esteem
24. Disturbed self-esteem
25. Chronic
26. Disturbed body image
27. 2. This often results from long-standing negative evaluations or feelings about the self.
28. 2. It is helpful to include people who have meaning to the client.
29. 1. Shock and disbelief is the first stage of the grieving process.
30. 3. It may help to talk to someone who has lived through and coped with the experience.
31. 4. Encouraging choices in care promotes a sense of power and control.
32. 1

Copyright © 2004, Elsevier Science (USA). All Rights Reserved.

33. 2
34. 3
35. 4
36. 3
37. 1

CHAPTER 41

1. e
2. d
3. a
4. b
5. f
6. c
7. T
8. T
9. T
10. F. Anxiety disorders are common.
11. T
12. T
13. F. It is a learned behavior that is a conditioned response to a specific stimulus.
14. T
15. T
16. F. A panic attack is sudden.
17. biological, ego
18. vulnerability
19. severe
20. pathological
21. obsession
22. Psychoanalytic
23. Powerlessness
24. environmental
25. obsessive, compulsive
26. economic
27. 2. *Powerlessness* is associated with a perceived lack of control over situations or life events.
28. 1. This is an early goal. The others would be achieved later.
29. 3. Active listening involves listening to feelings as well as words.
30. 4
31. 3
32. 4

CHAPTER 42

1. i
2. b
3. l
4. m
5. f
6. o

7. p
8. q
9. g
10. h
11. c
12. a
13. e
14. n
15. d
16. j
17. k
18. T
19. F. Low, not high, socioeconomic status is a factor.
20. T
21. T
22. F. Hope can be present.
23. T
24. T
25. risk, health
26. housing
27. Social status
28. Social
29. energy
30. control
31. self-determination
32. 4. Social needs are also concerned with the social or environmental structures, such as the assessment of the risk of neighborhood violence and neighborhood resources, affecting the client's life.
33. 2. Helping a person to have a sense of relatedness to others, such as helping her contact her parents, can instill hope.
34. 2. To evaluate interventions for *Hopelessness,* assess for a change in the way the person thinks about the self in relation to others, the environment, and the self.
35. 1
36. 4
37. 3
38. 1
39. 1

CHAPTER 43

1. c
2. g
3. h
4. i
5. b
6. f

7. e
8. d
9. a
10. T
11. T
12. T
13. F. This refers to an orthotist.
14. F. These are long-term care facilities.
15. T
16. T
17. F. This client would have unilateral neglect
18. injury, mental conditions
19. physical, bowel, skin
20. coping
21. Assisted
22. Americans, Disabilities
23. Functional Independence Measure
24. maximizing, complications
25. 2. The physical therapist assesses a client's range of motion, mobility, strength, balance, and gait.
26. 4. Respite care is a temporary service enabling informal caregivers to take a break.
27. 1. *Deficient self-care* is applicable to people experiencing impaired ability to perform any one of the basic self-care activities.
28. 2
29. 3
30. 3
31. 3
32. 4

CHAPTER 44

1. d
2. n
3. a
4. f
5. q
6. k
7. j
8. i
9. e
10. h
11. m
12. o
13. l
14. r
15. p

Copyright © 2004, Elsevier Science (USA). All Rights Reserved.

16. c
17. g
18. b
19. T
20. F. This is a result of dysfunctional grieving.
21. T
22. T
23. T
24. F. Many people experience these feelings of relief or emancipation.
25. F. This refers to the person who is uncomfortable facing the reality of his or her own death.
26. religious, condolences, burial
27. self
28. recognition
29. reflection
30. family
31. presence
32. Condemnation
33. 2. Recognition: shock and denial: somatic responses: These may include gastrointestinal symptoms and cardiopulmonary reactions.
34. 1. This is the act of choosing when and to whom a person will give attention to a loss and allow thoughts and feeling to enter the conscious mind.
35. 3. This is an unexpected, involuntary resurgence of acute grief-related emotions and behaviors triggered by routine events.
36. 2
37. 3
38. 4
39. 4

CHAPTER 45

1. f
2. m
3. j
4. b
5. c
6. e
7. h
8. q
9. i
10. o
11. n
12. l
13. p

14. d
15. a
16. g
17. k
18. T
19. F. Gender identity is an internal sense.
20. F. Sexual patterns may not precisely fit with prevailing expectations.
21. T
22. F. At least one third of nurses never assessed their client's sexual health.
23. T
24. T
25. biological, cultural
26. adolescence
27. Orgasm
28. emotional, love
29. embarrassment
30. sexual
31. touch
32. 1. The correct diagnosis is *Ineffective sexuality patterns:* the state in which an individual expresses concern regarding his or her sexuality.
33. 2. Because of the additional information about not having sexual relations with her husband for the last 3 months, the nurse should also consider the diagnosis of *Sexual dysfunction.*
34. 1. The first step in the PLISSIT model is *permission* to discuss sexual issues.
35. 1
36. 2
37. 2
38. 4
39. 1

CHAPTER 46

1. m
2. p
3. k
4. l
5. g
6. i
7. c
8. j
9. n
10. b
11. o

12. a
13. q
14. d
15. f
16. e
17. h
18. T
19. F. It is the exhaustion stage.
20. T
21. F. This refers to rationalization.
22. T
23. T
24. F. Stress is highly individualized.
25. F. This defines transference.
26. T
27. alarm reaction
28. crisis
29. developmental, situational
30. projection
31. genetics, developmental stage
32. sympathetic
33. coping
34. adulthood
35. denial
36. 2. He is drinking and does not acknowledge that his wound is infected.
37. 3. A therapeutic relationship is necessary to build trust and is a precursor to other interventions.
38. 4. Knowledge and control are best achieved by helping him learn how to manage his health status.
39. 1. Relaxation and music can be used together. The other methods are cognitive coping methods.
40. 2
41. 3
42. 1
43. 1

CHAPTER 47

1. k
2. n
3. g
4. t
5. s
6. p
7. q
8. a
9. i
10. d

Copyright © 2004, Elsevier Science (USA). All Rights Reserved.

11. r
12. h
13. m
14. j
15. e
16. l
17. c
18. f
19. o
20. b
21. T
22. T
23. F. This occurs in a healthy family.
24. T
25. T
26. F. Interventions may not remembered or may be rejected.
27. T
28. F. They are more likely to when they have inadequate support systems.
29. T
30. T
31. caregiver
32. affective, socialization, health
33. coping
34. trusting
35. ambivalent
36. stress
37. perception
38. insight
39. 2. An example of an extrafamily stressor is when a caregiver quits work to care for a family member and then experiences a financial hardship.
40. 1. She is vulnerable for felt difficulty in performing the family caregiver role.
41. 4. Providing direct assistance helps the caregiver identify professional resources.
42. 3
43. 4
44. 2
45. 3
46. 2
47. 4

CHAPTER 48

1. f
2. e

3. g
4. i
5. c
6. d
7. b
8. j
9. a
10. h
11. T
12. F. They are not necessarily synonymous.
13. F. Faith is belief without proof.
14. F. Nurses commonly avoid addressing spirituality.
15. T
16. T
17. T
18. God
19. Hope
20. Taoists
21. denominations
22. beliefs
23. spiritual
24. prayer
25. 2. Mexican-Americans have a tendency toward traditional values of family roles, including men heading the family.
26. 4. Asking a client "What has bothered you most about being sick?" helps you assess the client's perceived relation between spiritual beliefs and health.
27. 4. The diagnosis is *Spiritual distress*: disruption in the life principle that pervades a person's entire being and that integrates and transcends one's biological and psychological nature.
28. 4
29. 4
30. 2
31. 2
32. 4

CHAPTER 49

1. h
2. n
3. g
4. l
5. p
6. o

7. m
8. b
9. i
10. q
11. d
12. c
13. a
14. j
15. f
16. k
17. e
18. T
19. F. These are duties of the circulating nurse.
20. T
21. T
22. T
23. F. Pain is expected and normal.
24. T
25. T
26. F. The drug of choice is dantrolene sodium.
27. T
28. elective
29. preinduction
30. general
31. surgeon
32. standard
33. after
34. Laryngospasm
35. incentive spirometer
36. 6
37. Verbal, written
38. 1. *Anxiety* is expected due to the uncertain outcome of the surgery.
39. 3. They should be done ten to twelve times every 1 to 2 hours for best effect.
40. 2. It will help him prevent alveolar collapse and move secretions to large airway passages for easier expectoration.
41. 3. Splinting the incision makes movement more comfortable.
42. 4
43. 2
44. 3
45. 1
46. 4

Copyright © 2004, Elsevier Science (USA). All Rights Reserved.

Name _____ Specific Skill Performed _____

Date _____ Attempt Number _____

Instructor _____ PASS _____ FAIL _____

Performance Checklist 7–1: Assessing Temperature

	S	U	Comments
1. Correctly used aseptic technique and standard precautions.			
2. Appropriately prepared client.			
3. Selected an appropriate route and thermometer.			
4. Oral route with glass mercury-filled thermometer.			
a. Covered thermometer with sheath.			
b. Shook down mercury.			
c. Correctly placed thermometer under tongue.			
d. Correctly read temperature after 2-4 minutes.			
e. Correctly documented findings on graphic record.			
5. Rectal or axillary route with glass mercury-filled thermometer.			
a. Identified rationale for rectal or axillary route.			
b. Put on clean gloves.			
c. Shook down mercury. Used sheath lubricant for rectal route.			
d. Positioned client in left Sims' position and draped for rectal privacy.			
e. Inserted thermometer approximately 1.5 inches into rectum or axilla.			
f. Held thermometer in place for 2 to 4 minutes.			
g. Wiped down thermometer with tissue.			
h. Correctly read temperature.			
i. Converted rectal or axillary reading to oral equivalent.			
j. Correctly documented findings.			
6. Electronic thermometer including tympanic route.			
a. Removed probe (electronic) or turned on the unit (tympanic).			
b. Attached probe cover using aseptic technique.			
c. Placed thermometer or probe under client's tongue (electronic) or in external auditory canal (tympanic) until unit beeps.			
d. Correctly read temperature.			
e. Released probe cover using aseptic technique.			
f. Correctly documented findings.			

Additional Comments:

Copyright © 2004, Elsevier Science (USA). All Rights Reserved.

Name _____ Specific Skill Performed _____

Date _____ Attempt Number _____

Instructor _____ PASS _____ FAIL _____

Performance Checklist 7–2:   Assessing Radial and Apical Pulse

	S	U	Comments
Assessing Radial Pulse			
1. Placed client in a comfortable and relaxed position, such as with client's arm across abdomen.			
2. Located the radial artery using pads of middle fingers on inside of client's wrist.			
3. Compressed radial artery firmly against underlying bone and released pressure until pulse became palpable.			
4. Counted pulse accurately, also assessing quality and rhythm (for an appropriate length of time and within two beats of a partner's count).			
5. Documented findings.			
6. Identified reportable findings.			
Assessing Apical Pulse			
1. Positioned client supine or in other comfortable position. Provided for client privacy.			
2. Located the pulse at 5th intercostal space, mid-clavicular line.			
3. Placed diaphragm of stethoscope firmly against client's chest without rubbing against clothing or linen.			
4. Counted pulse accurately and noted rhythm (for 1 full minute and within two beats of a partner's count).			
5. Documented findings.			
6. Identified reportable findings.			
Assessing Apical/Radial Pulse			
1. Positioned client correctly. Provided for client privacy.			
2. Located the apical pulse correctly. Provided correct instructions to a partner who counts the radial pulse.			
3. Counted pulse accurately (for 1 minute and within two beats of a partner's count).			
4. Documented findings.			
5. Identified reportable findings.			

Additional Comments:

Copyright © 2004, Elsevier Science (USA). All Rights Reserved.

Name _____   Specific Skill Performed _____

Date _____   Attempt Number _____

Instructor _____   PASS _____ FAIL _____

Performance Checklist 7–3:   Assessing Respiration

		S	U	Comments
1.	Provided quiet, relaxed position (sitting or lying down) with client's anterior thorax easily visible and lungs having full ability for excursion.			
2.	Counted respirations unobserved by client for 30 seconds (regular rhythm) and then multiplied number by two. Counted for a full minute with an infant, child, or an adult who has an irregular rhythm.			
3.	Documented findings accurately on graphic record.			
4.	Identified reportable findings.			

Additional Comments:

Copyright © 2004, Elsevier Science (USA). All Rights Reserved.

Name _____   Specific Skill Performed _____

Date _____   Attempt Number _____

Instructor _____   PASS _____ FAIL _____

Performance Checklist 7–4:   Assessing Blood Pressure

	S	U	Comments
1. Selected correct size cuff (bladder fits almost completely around arm; width is about ⅔ the length of client's upper arm).			
2. Chose appropriate arm (no injury, shunt, burn, IV line, cast, breast or axillary surgery to that side).			
3. Placed arm level with heart, palm up, in a relaxed and comfortable position.			
4. Correctly applied the cuff to the client's arm.			
a. Was not placed over clothing.			
b. Bottom edge was 1 inch above antecubital fossa.			
c. Center of cuff was directly and snugly over brachial artery with space to place stethoscope.			
5. Positioned sphygmomanometer at eye level.			
6. Obtained palpatory blood pressure.			
a. Palpated brachial or radial pulse.			
b. Inflated cuff until pulse disappeared.			
c. Released pressure slowly until pulse returned.			
d. Noted reading and quickly released cuff.			
7. Obtained blood pressure reading.			
a. Waited 30 to 60 seconds after obtaining palpatory blood pressure.			
b. Placed bell of stethoscope lightly over brachial artery.			
c. Tightened screw clamp of cuff and quickly inflated to 30 mm Hg above palpatory blood pressure reading.			
d. Deflated cuff slowly at 2 to 3 mm/second, noting point at which a soft tapping Korotkoff sound was heard (systolic reading).			
e. Continued deflating cuff slowly until sound became muffled (children) or stopped (adult), noting this as the diastolic reading.			
8. Read the blood pressure within 4 mm Hg of a partner's simultaneous reading using dual stethoscope.			
9. Documented findings in graphic record.			
10. Identified reportable findings.			

Additional Comments:

Copyright © 2004, Elsevier Science (USA). All Rights Reserved.

Name _____   Specific Skill Performed _____

Date _____   Attempt Number _____

Instructor _____   PASS _____ FAIL _____

Performance Checklist 20–1: Administering Oral Medications

		S	U	Comments
1.	Verified order and client allergies. Assessed appropriate parameters (e.g., blood pressure, pulse) if applicable.			
2.	Dispensed solid medication correctly.			
	a. Selected medication, calculated dose based on labeled concentration, and rechecked dose.			
	b. Placed medication into soufflé cup if whole tablet used, or split a scored tablet with a gloved hand or cutting device for a partial dose.			
	c. Left unit-dose medications in original container and placed all in a single cup, except for medications requiring special assessments.			
	d. Removed tablet from stock medication bottle by dropping it into bottle cap and transferring to soufflé cup.			
3.	Dispensed liquid medication correctly.			
	a. Poured liquid dose by mixing medication and removing lid, placing it upside down.			
	b. Held bottle with label under palm of hand.			
	c. Poured dose holding plastic cup at eye level with thumbnail at dose mark and used bottom of the meniscus as measuring guide.			
	d. Wiped lip of container before closing.			
4.	Rechecked all medications and dosages after dispensing.			
5.	Identified client using identification bracelet or asking client to state name, and performed final assessments.			
6.	Gave medications to client.			
	a. Rechecked accuracy of medication that client questioned.			
	b. Removed unit-dose wrappers and placed medications in cup or client's hand per client preference.			
	c. Offered sufficient liquid for swallowing and ensured that client swallowed all medications.			
7.	Documented medications administered immediately and stated to check client response in 30 minutes.			

Additional Comments:

Copyright © 2004, Elsevier Science (USA). All Rights Reserved.

Name _____ Specific Skill Performed _____

Date _____ Attempt Number _____

Instructor _____ PASS _____ FAIL _____

Performance Checklist 20–2: Withdrawing Medication from an Ampule

	S	U	Comments
1. Opened ampule by tapping upper chamber to drop fluid into lower chamber.			
2. Wrapped alcohol swab or gauze pad around ampule neck and snapped neck so it opened away from nurse.			
3. Placed ampule on flat surface and withdrew medication into syringe without touching needle against ampule rim.			
4. Tilted ampule as needed to keep needle below level of medication. Did not inject air into ampule.			
5. Ejected excess air or fluid from syringe.			
6. Recapped needle and replaced with new one, properly discarding old needle.			
7. Compared final volume to dose ordered.			

Additional Comments:

Copyright © 2004, Elsevier Science (USA). All Rights Reserved.

Name _____   Specific Skill Performed _____

Date _____   Attempt Number _____

Instructor _____   PASS _____ FAIL _____

Performance Checklist 20–3:   Withdrawing Medication from a Vial

	S	U	Comments
1. Removed plastic cap of new vial or wiped rubber seal of open one with alcohol swab. Used previously used vial only if opened within 30 days.			
2. Prepared syringe by securing capped needle to syringe with twisting motion and removed needle cover.			
3. Drew back on plunger to fill syringe with volume of air equal to the medication dose.			
4. Withdrew medication.			
a. Inserted needle into center of rubber seal and injected air.			
b. Inverted vial and withdrew medication slowly while holding vial at eye level. Kept tip of needle in solution at all times.			
c. Removed excess air by tapping side of syringe with finger and pushed air back into vial. Removed additional fluid if needed to obtain correct dose.			
d. Returned vial to upright position and removed needle by pulling back on barrel, not plunger. Removed excess air.			
5. Recapped needle and replaced with a new one if indicated.			
6. Compared volume of fluid in syringe with ordered dose.			

Additional Comments:

Copyright © 2004, Elsevier Science (USA). All Rights Reserved.

Name _____   Specific Skill Performed _____

Date _____   Attempt Number _____

Instructor _____   PASS _____ FAIL _____

Performance Checklist 20–4:   Mixing Insulin in a Single Syringe

	S	U	Comments
1. Mixed insulin in suspension by rotating vial between palms of hands.			
2. Wiped vials with alcohol after checking expiration dates.			
3. Added air to both vials.			
a. Drew up volume of air equal to dose of modified (NPH) insulin and injected into NPH vial without letting needle touch solution.			
b. Removed needle from vial.			
c. Drew up volume of air equal to dose of regular (unmodified) insulin and injected into regular insulin vial. Left needle in vial.			
4. Removed insulin from both vials.			
a. Inverted regular insulin vial and withdrew correct dose without air bubbles present.			
b. Turned vial upright and removed needle from vial.			
c. Cleansed port of NPH vial and inserted needle.			
d. Inverted vial and withdrew correct dose.			
e. Turned vial upright again and removed needle. Recapped using scoop technique.			
5. Had another licensed nurse double-check the dose.			
6. Administered within 5 minutes of preparation.			

Additional Comments:

Copyright © 2004, Elsevier Science (USA). All Rights Reserved.

Name _____   Specific Skill Performed _____

Date _____   Attempt Number _____

Instructor _____   PASS _____ FAIL _____

Performance Checklist 20–5:   Administering an Intradermal Injection

	S	U	Comments
1. Checked order and noted client allergies.			
2. Withdrew medication from vial and brought dose to bedside.			
3. Prepared client for injection.			
a. Checked client identity.			
b. Explained procedure and placed client in proper position.			
c. Donned disposable gloves.			
4. Prepared injection site and syringe.			
a. Chose an area free from bruises, redness, or lesions.			
b. Cleansed skin with alcohol wipe using circular motion outward from injection site.			
c. Removed needle cap and checked that syringe was free of air and volume was correct.			
5. Injected medication.			
a. Held syringe in dominant hand and spread skin taut with nondominant hand.			
b. Inserted needle bevel-up at a 10 to 15 degree angle into skin for $\frac{1}{8}$-inch or until bevel disappeared from view. Needle was visible below skin surface and resistance was felt.			
c. Injected medication slowly while watching for wheal formation. If none appeared, withdrew needle slightly and continued injecting.			
d. Withdrew needle at same angle and used gauze pad to pat dry without rubbing.			
6. Observed for immediate allergic reaction.			
7. Disposed of equipment, removed gloves, and performed hand hygiene.			
8. Circled skin site and documented appropriately in medical record.			

Additional Comments:

Copyright © 2004, Elsevier Science (USA). All Rights Reserved.

Name _____   Specific Skill Performed _____

Date _____   Attempt Number _____

Instructor _____   PASS _____ FAIL _____

Performance Checklist 20–6: Administering a Subcutaneous (SC) Injection

	S	U	Comments
1. Checked order, noting any client allergies.			
2. Withdrew medication correctly and brought materials to bedside.			
3. Prepared client.			
a. Checked client identity.			
b. Explained procedure.			
c. Placed client in proper position.			
d. Donned disposable gloves.			
4. Prepared injection site and syringe.			
a. Chose an area free from bruises, redness, or lesions.			
b. Cleansed skin with alcohol wipe using circular motion outward from injection site.			
c. Removed needle cap and checked that syringe was free of air and volume was correct.			
5. Injected the medication.			
a. Held syringe in dominant hand between thumb and forefinger.			
b. Pinched or "bunched up" SC tissue between thumb and forefinger of nondominant hand.			
c. Quickly inserted needle up to hub at 45- or 90-degree angle, depending on needle length.			
d. Released tissue and grasped distal end of syringe. Aspirated for blood return unless injecting insulin or heparin.			
e. Injected medication slowly and steadily if no blood return. Discarded syringe and repeated procedure if positive blood return.			
f. Withdrew needle at same angle used for insertion and massaged area with alcohol swab unless heparin given.			
6. Disposed of equipment, removed gloves, and performed hand hygiene.			
7. Documented appropriately and stated to recheck client in 30 minutes.			

Additional Comments:

Copyright © 2004, Elsevier Science (USA). All Rights Reserved.

Name _____   Specific Skill Performed _____

Date _____   Attempt Number _____

Instructor _____   PASS _____ FAIL _____

Performance Checklist 20–7:   Administering an Intramuscular Injection

	S	U	Comments
1. Checked order, noting any client allergies.			
2. Withdrew medication correctly and brought materials to bedside.			
3. Prepared client.			
a. Checked client identity.			
b. Explained procedure.			
c. Placed client in proper position.			
d. Donned clean disposable gloves.			
4. Prepared injection site and syringe.			
a. Chose an area free from bruises, redness, or lesions.			
b. Cleansed skin with alcohol wipe using circular motion outward from injection site.			
c. Removed needle cap and checked that syringe was free of air and volume was correct.			
5. Injected medication.			
a. Held syringe in dominant hand between thumb and forefinger.			
b. Spread skin taut between thumb and forefinger of nondominant hand, or displaced tissue using Z-track technique.			
c. Inserted needle quickly at 90-degree angle up to hub.			
d. Released skin unless using Z-track technique and grasped distal end of syringe in nondominant hand.			
e. Aspirated for blood return by pulling back gently on plunger with thumb and forefinger of dominant hand. Discarded syringe and began procedure again if blood seen.			
f. Injected medication slowly at a rate of about 10 seconds per mL.			
g. Waited a few seconds, withdrew needle quickly at same angle used for injection. Applied gentle pressure to site with alcohol wipe or small gauze.			
6. Disposed of equipment, removed gloves, and performed hand hygiene.			
7. Documented appropriately and stated to recheck client at appropriate time interval.			

Additional Comments:

Copyright © 2004, Elsevier Science (USA). All Rights Reserved.

Name _____   Specific Skill Performed _____

Date _____   Attempt Number _____

Instructor _____   PASS _____ FAIL _____

Performance Checklist 20–8:   Adding Medication to an IV Bag

	S	U	Comments
1. Checked medication order.			
2. Drew up medication correctly into a syringe from vial or ampule.			
3. Injected medication into IV solution.			
a. Closed roller clamp on tubing if already attached to solution bag.			
b. Wiped medication port of IV bag with alcohol wipe.			
c. Inserted needle into center of medication port and injected medication into bag.			
d. Withdrew needle and properly disposed of needle-syringe assembly without recapping.			
e. Rotated solution bag gently but thoroughly.			
f. Affixed a medication label to bag with medication name, dose, date, time, and nurse's initials noted.			
4. Primed tubing and hung solution according to standard procedure.			
5. Documented appropriately.			

Additional Comments:

Copyright © 2004, Elsevier Science (USA). All Rights Reserved.

Name _____   Specific Skill Performed _____

Date _____   Attempt Number _____

Instructor _____   PASS _____ FAIL _____

Performance Checklist 20–9:   Administering an IV Medication by Intermittent Infusion

	S	U	Comments
1. Checked order and prepared and labeled IV medication.			
2. Administered IV medication through an existing IV line.			
a. Attached secondary tubing to IV bag using standard protocol. Ensured that nonvented tubing was attached to IV bag and vented tubing was attached to IV bottle. Primed and labeled bag, as appropriate, and brought materials to bedside.			
b. Identified client, assessed IV site, and donned gloves if part of agency policy.			
c. Removed cap from distal IV tubing and attached needle or needleless device.			
d. Wiped IV additive port of primary IV line with alcohol swab and attached secondary IV tubing to primary line above the level of the regulator clamp.			
e. Lowered primary IV solution below level of the IV medication bag using hook provided by manufacturer. Opened roller clamp on secondary tubing or regulated IV medication drip rate or set infusion pump as ordered. Returned to reset drip rate if needed and reassessed client.			
3. Administered IV medication through a heparin lock (intermittent infusion device).			
a. Attached tubing as needed to IV medication bag or bottle using standard protocol. Primed tubing and attached needle or needleless device.			
b. Withdrew 3 mL sterile normal saline solution into 3 mL syringe (vary amount according to policy) and brought all materials to bedside.			
c. Identified client, assessed IV site, and donned gloves if part of agency policy.			
d. Wiped port of intermittent infusion device with alcohol swab. Assessed site and flushed infusion port with sterile saline per protocol.			
e. Wiped port again. Attached IV medication tubing to infusion port and regulated flow rate.			
f. Returned upon completion of infusion, closed roller clamp, removed tubing from port, and flushed again with ordered solution.			
4. Assessed IV site and client response and documented.			

Additional Comments:

Copyright © 2004, Elsevier Science (USA). All Rights Reserved.

Name _____ Specific Skill Performed _____

Date _____ Attempt Number _____

Instructor _____ PASS _____ FAIL _____

Performance Checklist 20–10: Administering an IV Push Medication

	S	U	Comments
1. Checked medication order and assessed client allergies. Prepared medication and brought materials to bedside.			
2. Checked client identity, assessed IV site, and donned gloves if part of agency policy.			
3. Administered medication through existing IV line.			
a. With alcohol swab, wiped IV additive port of primary line nearest to client.			
b. Inserted needle into port and pinched off tubing above injection port.			
c. Injected medication at manufacturer's recommended rate, using watch with second hand to time the injection.			
d. Released tubing, removed syringe, and assessed client tolerance of medication.			
4. Administered medication through an intermittent infusion device.			
a. Drew up normal saline into two syringes in a volume according to agency policy (often 3 mL). Labeled syringes.			
b. Wiped port of intermittent infusion device with alcohol swab.			
c. Inserted one syringe with normal saline and injected slowly. Removed needle and syringe.			
d. Wiped port again with alcohol swab. Inserted syringe with medication into port and injected at manufacturer's recommended rate. Used watch with second hand to ensure accurate timing. Assessed site during injection.			
e. Wiped port again with alcohol swab. Inserted second normal saline flush syringe into port and injected slowly. Withdrew needle and syringe and correctly disposed of all supplies.			
5. Documented medication according to policy.			

Additional Comments:

Copyright © 2004, Elsevier Science (USA). All Rights Reserved.

Name _____   Specific Skill Performed _____

Date _____   Attempt Number _____

Instructor _____   PASS _____ FAIL _____

Performance Checklist 20–11:   Administering an Eye Medication

	S	U	Comments
1. Checked medication order and noted any client allergies.			
2. Prepared client for medication instillation.			
a. Checked client's identity and explained procedure.			
b. Donned clean gloves, and hyperextended client's head.			
c. Assessed condition of eye and washed away exudate, wiping from inner to outer canthus.			
3. Administered eye drop.			
a. Removed cap and filled medicine dropper (if used) to prescribed amount.			
b. Placed nondominant hand on client's cheekbone under eyelid and pulled downward against bony orbit to expose lower conjunctival sac. Held tissue or cotton ball under eyelid and applied slight pressure to inner canthus.			
c. Rested dominant hand against client's forehead and held medication $\frac{1}{2}$ to $\frac{3}{4}$ of an inch above conjunctival sac.			
d. Asked client to look up at ceiling and instilled prescribed number of drops into lower conjunctival sac.			
e. Asked client to gently close eye and move it around.			
f. Applied gentle pressure over lacrimal duct for one minute or asked client to do so.			
4. Administered eye ointment.			
a. Removed cap from tube and placed on its side. Squeezed and discarded small bead of medication.			
b. Separated client's eyelids with thumb and forefinger of nondominant hand, pulling lower eyelid over bony prominence of cheek (or drew upper lid up and away from eyeball if instilling in upper lid).			
c. Asked client to look up for instillation in lower lid (down for instillation in upper) and applied thin layer of ointment along inside edge of lower or upper lid, moving from inner to outer canthus.			
d. Asked client to gently close eye and move it around.			
5. Administered eye disk.			
a. Opened package and pressed tip of index finger against convex part of disk.			
b. Pulled lower eyelid away from eye with nondominant hand and asked client to look up.			

Copyright © 2004, Elsevier Science (USA). All Rights Reserved.

		S	U	Comments
c.	Placed disk horizontally in conjunctival sac between iris and lower lid.			
d.	Pulled lower lid out, up and over disk. Asked client to blink a few times. Repeated if still visible.			
e.	Had client place fingers against closed lids and press without rubbing eyes or moving disk.			
f.	Removed disk by inverting lower eyelid to see disk. Used thumb and index finger of dominant hand to pinch disk and lift it from conjunctival sac. Stroked closed eyelid with fingertip in gentle, long, circular motions to lower a disk caught in the upper eye.			
6.	Removed gloves, performed hand hygiene, and documented correctly.			

Additional Comments:

Copyright © 2004, Elsevier Science (USA). All Rights Reserved.

Name _____   Specific Skill Performed _____

Date _____   Attempt Number _____

Instructor _____   PASS _____ FAIL _____

Performance Checklist 20–12:   Irrigating an Eye

	S	U	Comments
1. Prepared client for irrigation.			
a. Helped client sit or lie with head tilted toward eye to be irrigated.			
b. Used water-proof pad and gloves.			
c. Poured irrigating solution into container and drew up into syringe using aseptic technique.			
d. Cleaned eyelids and eyelashes with cotton ball moistened with solution or normal saline.			
e. Positioned curved basin under cheek and asked client to hold if possible.			
2. Irrigated eye.			
a. Used nondominant hand to hold client's upper lid open and expose lower conjunctival sac.			
b. Held irrigation syringe 1 inch above eye without touching eye and pushed fluid gently into conjunctival sac, directing flow from inner canthus to outer canthus.			
c. Repeated irrigation until secretions and irrigating solution were gone. Allowed client to close eyes intermittently during procedure.			
d. Dried area with cotton balls and offered client a towel to dry face and neck.			
3. Removed gloves, performed hand hygiene, and documented correctly.			

Additional Comments:

Copyright © 2004, Elsevier Science (USA). All Rights Reserved.

Name _____   Specific Skill Performed _____

Date _____   Attempt Number _____

Instructor _____   PASS _____ FAIL _____

Performance Checklist 20–13:   Administering an Ear Medication

	S	U	Comments
1. Checked the medication order and any client allergies.			
2. Prepared client for medication instillation.			
a. Checked client's identity.			
b. Explained procedure and helped client to lie with affected ear upward.			
c. Donned clean gloves.			
d. Assessed condition of ear and washed away cerumen or exudates with cotton-tipped applicators.			
3. Administered medication.			
a. Removed cap from bottle and placed cap on its side. Filled medication dropper to prescribed amount.			
b. Pulled the pinna up and back for an adult or down and back for a child.			
c. Held dropper $\frac{1}{2}$ of an inch above ear canal and instilled ordered number of drops.			
d. Asked client to maintain side-lying position for 2 to 3 minutes.			
e. Used finger to apply gentle pressure to tragus of ear or asked client to do so.			
f. Placed a cotton ball into outermost portion of ear canal.			
4. Removed gloves, performed hand hygiene, and documented correctly.			
5. Stated to check on client in 15 minutes to remove cotton ball, assess condition, and reposition.			

Additional Comments:

Copyright © 2004, Elsevier Science (USA). All Rights Reserved.

Name _____   Specific Skill Performed _____

Date _____   Attempt Number _____

Instructor _____   PASS _____ FAIL _____

Performance Checklist 20–14:   Administering an Intranasal Medication

	S	U	Comments
1. Checked medication order and noted any client allergies.			
2. Prepared client.			
a. Checked identity of client.			
b. Explained procedure.			
c. Donned clean gloves.			
d. Asked client to blow nose unless contraindicated.			
3. Administered nasal spray medication.			
a. Removed cap from bottle and placed cap on its side.			
b. Asked adult client to tilt head backward and supported head with nondominant hand. Kept a child's head in upright position.			
c. Held medication container just inside tip of nostril without touching nasal tissue.			
d. Asked client to occlude other nostril and inhale while spraying in.			
e. Positioned client for comfort.			
4. Administered nasal drops.			
a. Removed cap from bottle and placed cap on its side.			
b. Positioned client to accommodate intended site of action. Supported head with nondominant hand.			
c. Held tip of dropper just above intended nostril and pointed toward midline of ethmoid bone.			
d. Instilled ordered number of drops with client breathing through mouth, and without touching nasal tissue with dropper.			
e. Asked client to maintain head position for 5 minutes and then assisted to comfortable position.			
5. Removed gloves, performed hand hygiene, and documented correctly.			

Additional Comments:

Copyright © 2004, Elsevier Science (USA). All Rights Reserved.

Name _____   Specific Skill Performed _____

Date _____   Attempt Number _____

Instructor _____   PASS _____ FAIL _____

Performance Checklist 20–15:   Administering a Vaginal Medication

	S	U	Comments
1. Checked medication order.			
2. Prepared client for medication instillation.			
a. Identified client.			
b. Explained procedure and offered opportunity to void.			
c. Provided privacy and assisted client to supine position with abdomen and legs draped.			
d. Donned clean gloves, inspected area, and provided hygiene as needed.			
3. Administered vaginal suppository.			
a. Removed suppository from wrapper and inserted into applicator, if used.			
b. Lubricated rounded end with water-soluble lubricant. Lubricated index finger of gloved dominant hand if not using applicator.			
c. Separated client's labia with nondominant hand and inserted rounded end of suppository along posterior vaginal wall for entire finger length.			
d. Withdrew finger or applicator and wiped away excess lubricant from client's genitals.			
4. Administered a foam, jelly, or cream medication.			
a. Filled applicator with medication per package directions.			
b. Separated labia with nondominant hand, pointed applicator toward client's sacrum and used dominant hand to insert applicator 2 to 3 inches into vagina.			
c. Depressed plunger on applicator to push medication out of applicator.			
d. Withdrew applicator and placed it on tissue or paper towel.			
e. Wiped away excess medication from genitals.			
5. Assisted client to comfortable position and asked her to remain supine for 5 to 10 minutes.			
6. Offered perineal pad if needed.			
7. Washed applicator with soap and water and stored for future use.			
8. Removed gloves, performed hand hygiene, and documented.			

Additional Comments:

Copyright © 2004, Elsevier Science (USA). All Rights Reserved.

Name _____   Specific Skill Performed _____

Date _____   Attempt Number _____

Instructor _____   PASS _____ FAIL _____

Performance Checklist 20–16:   Administering a Rectal Medication

	S	U	Comments
1. Checked medication order.			
2. Prepared client for medication instillation.			
a. Identified client.			
b. Explained procedure and offered opportunity to void.			
c. Assisted client to left lateral Sims' position with upper leg flexed, and draped client for privacy.			
d. Donned clean gloves, inspected area, and provided hygiene as needed.			
3. Administered medication using clean aseptic technique.			
a. Removed suppository from packaging. Lubricated rounded end of suppository and index finger of gloved, dominant hand.			
b. Instructed client to breathe slowly and deeply through mouth.			
c. Separated buttocks with gloved, nondominant hand.			
d. Used dominant hand to insert rounded end of suppository 4 inches into rectal canal along rectal wall (2 inches for child).			
e. Withdrew finger and wiped away any fecal material or excess lubricant from client's anus.			
f. Asked client to remain on side for 5 to 30 minutes depending on medication.			
4. Removed gloves, performed hand hygiene, and gave client call bell to ring when urge to defecate was felt.			
5. Returned after 5 minutes to see if suppository was expelled (reinserted if it was expelled). Assisted client as needed. Documented administration and results.			

Additional Comments:

Copyright © 2004, Elsevier Science (USA). All Rights Reserved.

Name _____   Specific Skill Performed _____

Date _____   Attempt Number _____

Instructor _____   PASS _____ FAIL _____

Performance Checklist 21–1:   Hand-Washing

	S	U	Comments
1. Turned on warm water faucet, wet hands, and lowered arms under running water with hands held lower than elbows.			
2. Used soap to rub all surfaces of hands, including palms, back of hands, and wrists. Worked soap into foamy lather while rubbing hands together using circular motions.			
3. Used care between fingers, creases, and breaks in skin, and under nails. Spent at least 15 to 30 seconds cleaning each hand.			
4. Rinsed hands with warm running water, with water washing down hands and over fingertips.			
5. Dried hands thoroughly with towel.			
6. If sink not foot-operated, used towel to turn off faucet, and discarded towel in receptacle.			

Additional Comments:

Copyright © 2004, Elsevier Science (USA). All Rights Reserved.

Performance Checklist 21–2:   Caring for a Client in Isolation

	S	U	Comments
Application of Barriers			
1. Performed hand hygiene.			
2. Picked up gown by collar and allowed it to unfold without touching floor.			
3. Put arms through sleeves and pulled gown up over shoulders.			
4. Fastened neckties and waist ties, making sure gown lapped over itself at back.			
5. Put on disposable gloves by pulling cuff of each glove over edge of gown sleeve, and interlaced fingers as needed to adjust fit of gloves.			
6. Donned mask by positioning over nose and mouth. Bent nose bar over bridge of nose, and fastened it in place with elastic or strings.			
7. Put on goggles, if indicated, after mask was in place.			
Removal of Barriers			
1. Without touching face or hair, removed goggles first next to receptacle at entrance to client's room. Untied gown at waist only.			
2. Removed gloves.			
a. Grasped outside cuff of one glove and pulled glove inside out over hand.			
b. Held removed glove in second hand, and pulled second glove off inside out over first.			
3. Removed gown.			
a. Untied gown at neck and allowed it to fall forward from shoulders.			
b. Slid hands through sleeves and removed them without touching outside of gown.			
c. Held gown at inside shoulder seams away from body, turned it inside out and folded it with contaminated side to the inside.			
d. Discarded in proper receptacle.			
4. Removed mask by pulling elastic or untying strings without touching outside surface. Discarded mask.			
5. Performed hand hygiene.			

Additional Comments:

Copyright © 2004, Elsevier Science (USA). All Rights Reserved.

Name _____   Specific Skill Performed _____

Date _____   Attempt Number _____

Instructor _____   PASS _____ FAIL _____

Performance Checklist 21–3:   Donning and Removing Sterile Gloves

	S	U	Comments
Donning Sterile Gloves			
1. Performed hand hygiene and removed rings with stones or irregular surfaces.			
2. Grasped package at tabs above sealed edge, peeled down, and discarded outer wrapper.			
3. Opened inner package.			
a. Placed inner package on flat surface, opened inner package at first fold, touched outside of folded edge and pulled outward.			
b. Opened next fold, pulling edge outward without touching inside of package.			
4. Put on first glove.			
a. Grasped folded edge of cuff of one glove.			
b. Lifted glove above wrapper and away from body.			
c. Slid opposite hand into glove. Did not adjust cuff or fingers at this time or let ungloved hand touch outside of glove.			
5. Put on second glove.			
a. Picked up second glove by sliding sterile gloved fingers under cuff edge. Kept gloved thumb off cuff of second glove.			
b. Slid fingers of opposite hand into glove. Let go of edge when hand in glove.			
c. Adjusted for comfort and fit.			
Removing Sterile Gloves			
1. Grasped outside of one glove near base of thumb and removed it by pulling inside out.			
2. Discarded glove or held it in palm of gloved hand.			
3. Slid ungloved thumb or fingers inside second glove and removed pulling it inside out.			
4. Discarded into appropriate receptacle and performed hand hygiene.			

Additional Comments:

Copyright © 2004, Elsevier Science (USA). All Rights Reserved.

Name _____ Specific Skill Performed _____

Date _____ Attempt Number _____

Instructor _____ PASS _____ FAIL _____

Performance Checklist 21–4:   Preparing a Sterile Field by Opening a Tray Wrapped in a Sterile Drape

	S	U	Comments
1. Performed hand hygiene and removed kit from outer wrapper.			
2. Positioned inner package in center of work surface with outer flap facing away from individual.			
3. Reached around (not over) package to open flap away from individual, touching outside of flap only.			
4. Opened side flaps one at a time, uppermost side first, and in same manner as first. Did not let hands move over sterile field.			
5. Opened innermost flap last and stood back far enough throughout procedure to avoid touching individual while opening.			

Additional Comments:

Copyright © 2004, Elsevier Science (USA). All Rights Reserved.

Name _____   Specific Skill Performed _____

Date _____   Attempt Number _____

Instructor _____   PASS _____ FAIL _____

Performance Checklist 21–5: Preparing a Sterile Field Using a Sterile Drape

	S	U	Comments
1. Established clean, dry, flat work area at waist level and close to client.			
2. Checked expiration date on supplies and checked for integrity of all packages.			
3. Set up a drape on a surface at least 2 inches larger on all sides than area needed to work with supplies.			
a. Opened outer wrapping of sterile cloth drape and kept drape sterile.			
b. Picked up drape by loose corner edge and lifted drape up and away from body.			
c. With other hand, grasped another corner edge and spread drape in air.			
d. Decided which surface should remain sterile and spread drape on table with sterile side facing up.			
4. Added dry sterile supplies.			
a. Opened peel-apart package by grasping edges designed to peel open.			
b. Opened package over sterile field so material fell freely from package onto field without touching the hands.			
c. Opened a wrapped package by holding object in one hand or by underside of wrapping.			
d. Unwrapped first corner away from body, then each side, then opened last corner toward body.			
e. Stabilized corners against wrist, turned object onto sterile field and dropped it onto field without touching sterile field.			
5. Added sterile liquids.			
a. Removed or loosened cap without touching inside of cap or rim of bottle.			
b. Placed cap face up on flat surface. Labeled bottle with date and time if first use.			
c. Donned sterile glove and arranged cup to hold liquid in upright position.			
d. Picked up liquid with ungloved hand so label was in palm of hand. Lipped bottle if not first use.			
e. Held bottle of solution 10 cm (4 inches) above container. Poured without spills or splashes. Avoided touching field with bottle lid.			
f. Replaced lid.			
g. Donned second sterile glove.			

Additional Comments:

Copyright © 2004, Elsevier Science (USA). All Rights Reserved.

Name _____   Specific Skill Performed _____

Date _____   Attempt Number _____

Instructor _____   PASS _____ FAIL _____

Performance Checklist 21–6:   Performing a Surgical Hand Scrub

		S	U	Comments
1.	Applied surgical attire (shoe covers, cap or hood, face mask, protective eyewear).			
2.	Opened scrub brush for ready use. Turned on water using control lever.			
3.	Wet hands and arms, keeping elbows flexed with hands higher than elbows, and allowing water to flow off arms at elbows.			
4.	Used plastic nail stick to clean under all fingernails.			
5.	Removed scrub brush from wrapper and wet it. Applied antimicrobial liquid if not contained in brush.			
6.	Scrubbed nails of one hand with 15 strokes and repeated with other hand. Scrubbed palm of one hand, each side of thumbs and fingers, and back of hand with 10 strokes each. Repeated for other hand.			
7.	Divided arms mentally into thirds, and scrubbed each third with 10 strokes or by time according to agency policy. Discarded brush.			
8.	Flexed arms and rinsed each arm from fingertips to elbow in a single smooth motion, letting water run off at elbows.			
9.	Released water control and walked backward into opening room with hands elevated in front and away from body.			
10.	Picked up sterile towel from sterile set-up area without dripping water onto field. Used one end of the towel to dry one hand using rotating motion and moving from fingers to elbow.			
11.	Used other end of towel to repeat with other hand. Discarded towel into designated area.			

Additional Comments:

Copyright © 2004, Elsevier Science (USA). All Rights Reserved.

Name _____   Specific Skill Performed _____

Date _____   Attempt Number _____

Instructor _____   PASS _____ FAIL _____

Performance Checklist 21–7:   Donning a Sterile Gown and Closed Gloving

	S	U	Comments
1. Donned surgical attire and scrubbed while designated person opened sterile gown and gloves.			
2. Donned gown.			
a. Identified inner surface of gown and picked it up beneath neckband without touching sterile field or outer surface of gown.			
b. Ensured control of all folded layers.			
c. Moved away from table, held gown away from body at arm's length, and allowed it to unfold from top down without touching floor.			
d. Held gown below neckband near shoulders and slid both hands into sleeves until fingers were at end of cuffs but not through them.			
e. Had someone tie gown.			
3. Donned first sterile glove.			
a. With hands covered by sterile gown cuffs, opened inner sterile glove package and picked up first glove by cuff.			
b. Positioned glove on forearm of dominant hand so cuff faced hand and fingers faced elbow.			
c. Began to put opposite hand into glove. Held cuff edge of glove with sleeve cover of hand to be gloved. Grasped back of glove cuff with sleeve-covered second hand and turned cuff over sleeve.			
d. Pushed fingers into glove.			
4. Donned second sterile glove.			
a. Used sterile hand to pick up second glove.			
b. Positioned and donned it in same manner as first.			
5. Adjusted both gloves for comfort and fit.			

Additional Comments:

Copyright © 2004, Elsevier Science (USA). All Rights Reserved.

Name _____ Specific Skill Performed _____

Date _____ Attempt Number _____

Instructor _____ PASS _____ FAIL _____

Performance Checklist 22–1: Using Protective Restraints

		S	U	Comments
1.	Assessed need for restraint, considered alternatives, and chose least restrictive restraint.			
2.	Applied restraint correctly.			
	a. Approached client and explained procedure in calm, reassuring manner.			
	b. If client did not understand need for restraint, proceeded by applying in gentle but firm manner.			
	c. Padded skin under restraint, especially over bony prominences.			
	d. Allowed room for two fingers to be inserted between restraint and limb to prevent circulatory constriction.			
	e. Avoided obstructing the client's breathing. Allowed freedom to turn in bed, if possible.			
	f. Used slipknot to tie restraint to bed frame rather than side rail. Did not tape a restraint note.			
	g. If out of bed, tied restraint in location accessible to staff but not accessible to client.			
3.	Took action to prevent complications.			
	a. Observed client, client's skin, and client's circulatory status every 30 minutes. Reoriented client with each contact.			
	b. Repositioned client, assessed respiratory status, and reassessed need for restraint every 2 hours.			
	c. Provided for food and fluid intake and toileting needs.			
4.	Documented properly: the rationale or behavior that lead to restraint, type and time of application, any going assessments and interventions, time of removal, and client response.			

Additional Comments:

Copyright © 2004, Elsevier Science (USA). All Rights Reserved.

Name _____   Specific Skill Performed _____

Date _____   Attempt Number _____

Instructor _____   PASS _____ FAIL _____

Performance Checklist 24–1:   Administering an Enteral Feeding

	S	U	Comments
1. Prepared client by ensuring comfort and privacy, and by raising head of bed 30 to 45 degrees. Performed hand hygiene.			
2. Assessed client.			
a. Listened to bowel sounds.			
b. Observed for abdominal distention or distress.			
c. Checked for reports or presence of diarrhea.			
3. Prepared for feeding.			
a. Selected formula at room temperature and checked expiration date.			
b. Donned clean gloves, confirmed tube placement by aspirating gastric contents, and checked amount of residual.			
c. Tested pH of gastric residual if ordered.			
4. Flushed tube with at least 50 mL of water using syringe with plunger removed. For small bore tubes, injected water slowly using syringe.			
5. Gave bolus feeding, verbalizing that it should take approximately 15 minutes.			
a. Using barrel of syringe as a funnel, filled barrel with feeding solution and let it instill by gravity.			
b. Refilled syringe when it drained to almost empty, and repeated until total dose given.			
c. Flushed with 50 mL water or other ordered amount.			
d. Clamped tube.			
e. Removed syringe, washed with tap water, and stored for future use.			
f. Covered tube with sterile gauze, and cleaned equipment.			
6. Gave an intermittent feeding.			
a. Flushed feeding tube with water and clamped tube.			
b. Primed feeding set with formula.			
c. Labeled new bag with time, date, and initials. Hung set from IV pole.			
d. Attached feeding set to feeding tube, and regulated flow rate so formula infused over 20 minutes.			
e. Clamped tube, removed feeding bag, cleaned bag with tap water, and stored equipment for future use.			

Copyright © 2004, Elsevier Science (USA). All Rights Reserved.

	S	U	Comments
7. Gave continuous feeding as outlined in steps 6a-c above, threaded tubing through infusion pump, and set pump at prescribed rate.			
8. Verbalized that medications given through feeding tube must be in liquid form or finely crushed.			
9. Cleaned feeding tube site.			
a. Verbalized to clean feeding tube site at least daily.			
b. Used clean technique and soap and water to clean area and dried area well.			
c. Observed for signs of infection.			
d. Applied dressing if ordered using split 4×4 gauze and non-allergenic tape.			
10. Verbalized to tape tube securely to gown, monitor client status, tidy environment, remove gloves, perform hand hygiene, and complete documentation.			

Additional Comments:

Copyright © 2004, Elsevier Science (USA). All Rights Reserved.

Performance Checklist 24–2:   Administering Parenteral Nutrition through a Central Line

	S	U	Comments
1. Confirmed physician order and checked order against listed ingredients on bag of solution and appearance.			
2. Checked the solution.			
a. Removed solution from refrigerator at least one hour before use.			
b. Observed solution for cloudiness, turbidity, particles, or cracks in container.			
c. Stated to return solution to pharmacy if lipid emulsion has separated from solution, giving an appearance of a brown layer.			
3. Assessed client (potassium, phosphorus, and glucose values, signs of inflammation or swelling at infusion site, frame of mind), and provided reassurance for any fears of procedural discomfort.			
4. Prepared solution and tubing.			
a. Connected infusion bag to IV tubing, filter, and extension tubing with clamps closed.			
b. Opened clamp, primed and reclamped tubing.			
c. Threaded tubing through infusion pump.			
d. Timed and dated new tubing.			
5. Prepared central line catheter and began infusion.			
a. Flushed catheter according to policy with saline.			
b. Donned sterile gloves.			
c. Cleaned catheter cap with alcohol.			
d. Used aseptic technique to insert needle or needleless connector into injection cap. Clamped tube or reminded client to perform Valsalva maneuver when accessing line or changing tubing.			
e. Unclamped tubing.			
f. Set infusion pump at prescribed rate. Verbalized to start flow rate slowly and monitor rate carefully.			
6. Verbalized not to use single-lumen line for blood sampling or blood infusion, to avoid adding medications to TPN solution at all times, and to avoid giving IV medications in same line if possible.			
7. Verbalized client parameters to monitor (VS, labs, weight, urine output, infusion site) and documentation to complete once infusion hung (date, time, client response, I & O). Removed gloves and performed hand hygiene.			

Additional Comments:

Copyright © 2004, Elsevier Science (USA). All Rights Reserved.

Name _____   Specific Skill Performed _____

Date _____   Attempt Number _____

Instructor _____   PASS _____ FAIL _____

Performance Checklist 25–1:   Inserting and Maintaining a Nasogastric Tube

	S	U	Comments
1. Performed hand hygiene and prepared the environment.			
a. Arranged all equipment on small table or bedside stand.			
b. Prepared clear occlusive dressing or cut tape (3-inch strip of 1-inch tape with $1\frac{1}{2}$-inch horizontal tear up center) to secure tube to nose after insertion.			
c. Checked suction apparatus and attached collection device and tubing; confirmed a pressure of 80 to 100 mm Hg when used for an adult.			
2. Prepared the client.			
a. Positioned client to enable swallowing, usually high Fowler's.			
b. Explained procedure and donned clean gloves.			
c. Assessed nostrils to determine which was best to use by inspecting for septal deviation, asking about history of broken nose, and occluding one nostril at a time and having client breathe through other nostril.			
3. Passed the tube.			
a. Measured length correctly (from client's nose to earlobe and then to xiphoid process).			
b. Marked length of tube to be passed with small piece of tape partially around tube and lubricated final 3 inches of tube.			
c. With head in neutral position, inserted tube through client's patent nostril and passed it to the nasopharynx.			
d. Asked client to bend head forward and sip water through straw while advancing tube into stomach.			
e. Checked placement by aspirating contents and checking pH (less than 5).			
f. Secured tube properly to nose.			
g. Connected nasogastric tube to suction tubing if ordered.			
h. Attached tube to gown with rubber band and safety pin, leaving slack to prevent accidental pulling on tube with head movement.			
i. Set suction to prescribed level.			
j. Removed gloves and performed hand hygiene.			
4. Documented procedure, findings, and client's tolerance.			
5. Described ongoing care and monitoring.			
a. Stated to provide comfort care to client's nose and mouth at least every 8 hours and as needed.			

Copyright © 2004, Elsevier Science (USA). All Rights Reserved.

		S	U	Comments
b.	Stated to inspect abdomen and auscultate bowel sounds at least every 8 hours.			
c.	Stated to monitor function of tube and document amount and characteristics of output, manifestations of fluid balance, electrolyte levels.			
d.	Stated to report excessive output (>100 mL/hr), total output that exceeds intake, bloody returns, or signs of fluid volume deficit.			
6. Irrigated tube.				
a.	Used a 50 to 60 mL irrigation syringe and 30 to 60 mL normal saline.			
b.	Correctly calculated intake and output, computing difference between amount instilled and amount aspirated back.			

Additional Comments:

Copyright © 2004, Elsevier Science (USA). All Rights Reserved.

Name _____   Specific Skill Performed _____

Date _____   Attempt Number _____

Instructor _____   PASS _____ FAIL _____

Performance Checklist 25–2: Removing a Nasogastric Tube

	S	U	Comments
1. Prepared client.			
a. Assessed client and determined presence of bowel sounds.			
b. Explained procedure.			
c. Placed emesis basin and opened plastic bag on table, donned clean gloves, and placed towel across client's chest.			
d. Turned off suction machine and disconnected nasogastric tube from suction tubing.			
e. Unpinned tube from client's gown or untaped it from cheek.			
f. Instilled 20 mL of air into tube to displace secretions back into client's stomach.			
g. Loosened tape on client's nose while holding distal end of tube.			
2. Removed tube.			
a. Instructed client to hold breath.			
b. Withdrew tube in one steady motion.			
c. Noted intactness of tip of the tube.			
d. Assisted with or provided mouth care.			
3. Documented findings and stated to continue to monitor bowel function.			

Additional Comments:

Copyright © 2004, Elsevier Science (USA). All Rights Reserved.

Name _____   Specific Skill Performed _____

Date _____   Attempt Number _____

Instructor _____   PASS _____ FAIL _____

Performance Checklist 25–3:   Initiating Peripheral Intravenous Therapy

	S	U	Comments
1. Prepared for IV therapy.			
a. Validated physician's order, client allergies, and checked for incompatibility between solutions or IV medications.			
b. Gathered supplies.			
c. Marked an IV time-tape strip and placed it on IV bag.			
d. Selected IV tubing and closed roller clamp.			
e. Removed protective covers on IV bag injection port and IV spike.			
f. Spiked IV bag; opened roller clamp and primed drip chamber ($\frac{1}{3}$ to $\frac{1}{2}$ full) and IV tubing; closed clamp.			
g. Labeled tubing with date, time, etc.			
h. Primed IV loop if used.			
2. Explained procedure and positioned client with arm below heart level.			
3. Identified and prepped site.			
a. Performed hand hygiene and donned clean gloves.			
b. Identified most distal vein possible and prepped skin (IV arm).			
c. Applied tourniquet at least 6 inches above projected site.			
d. Prepped skin using alcohol or povidone-iodine according to policy, starting at insertion point and wiping in an enlarging spiral (3-inch circle).			
e. Alternatively, used two pledgets, one using friction and multidirectional cleansing, and the second as described above.			
4. Inserted IV catheter.			
a. Removed needle or catheter from protective cover and held it bevel-up with dominant hand at 30-degree angle to skin, directly over or parallel to vein.			
b. Pierced through skin with one quick motion, decreasing the angle of needle or catheter to 15 degrees.			
c. Continued advancing until blood return obtained, then advanced another $\frac{1}{4}$ inch to be sure it is well into vein. (If needle is used, advanced until entire needle within vein).			
d. Released tourniquet.			
5. Attached primed IV tubing or attached primed saline lock device if ordered.			

Copyright © 2004, Elsevier Science (USA). All Rights Reserved.

Performance Checklist 25–3:   Initiating Peripheral Intravenous Therapy—cont'd

	S	U	Comments
6. Secured site.			
7. Dressed site with transparent dressing and stabilized tubing with additional piece of tape.			
8. Regulated flow of IV.			
a. Calculated drip rate correctly.			
b. Counted drops or set pump correctly.			
9. Documented procedure.			

Additional Comments:

Copyright © 2004, Elsevier Science (USA). All Rights Reserved.

Name _____ Specific Skill Performed _____

Date _____ Attempt Number _____

Instructor _____ PASS _____ FAIL _____

Performance Checklist 25–4: Discontinuing Peripheral Intravenous Therapy

	S	U	Comments
1. Prepared for procedure.			
a. Validated order and gathered equipment.			
b. Performed hand hygiene and donned clean gloves.			
c. Explained procedure to client.			
2. Removed catheter.			
a. Stopped flow of IV solution.			
b. Removed tape and dressing covering insertion site (tape may remain on catheter itself).			
c. Stabilized catheter and held alcohol swab or cotton gauze pledget over IV insertion site.			
d. Slid catheter out of vein and promptly applied pressure to site.			
e. Held pressure for 1 to 2 minutes until vein no longer leaked blood.			
f. Applied bandage (such as Band-aid) to site.			
3. Documented procedure.			

Additional Comments:

Copyright © 2004, Elsevier Science (USA). All Rights Reserved.

Name _____   Specific Skill Performed _____

Date _____   Attempt Number _____

Instructor _____   PASS _____ FAIL _____

Performance Checklist 25–5:   Changing the Dressing on a Central Line

	S	U	Comments
1. Prepared for procedure.			
a. Validated physician's order (or agency protocol).			
b. Performed hand hygiene, donned face mask and clean gloves.			
c. Explained procedure to client and assessed for allergy to povidone-iodine (Betadine).			
2. Removed soiled dressing.			
a. Opened tray and set up plastic trash bag.			
b. Removed soiled dressing in direction of insertion site with dominant hand while stabilizing central line device with nondominant hand.			
c. Held old dressing in dominant hand and used nondominant hand to pull glove of dominant hand over dressing.			
d. Removed other glove and discarded both in plastic bag. (Use reverse sequence if indicated by agency policy.)			
e. Performed hand hygiene.			
3. Cleaned the site.			
a. Set up sterile field.			
b. If kit available, donned sterile gloves and tore open Betadine and alcohol swabs.			
c. Started at site of IV access and used alcohol wipe to clean skin in circular motion outward 3 inches from insertion site. Repeated with two additional alcohol swabs.			
d. After alcohol evaporated (15 seconds), repeated cleansing with three Betadine swabs.			
4. Dressed site.			
a. Applied gauze (if used) and taped according to policy.			
b. Alternatively, applied transparent occlusive dressing so that IV access device was in center of dressing.			
c. Labeled dressing with date and time.			
5. Documented procedure.			

Additional Comments:

Name _____   Specific Skill Performed _____

Date _____   Attempt Number _____

Instructor _____   PASS _____ FAIL _____

Performance Checklist 26–1:   Irrigating a Wound

	S	U	Comments
1. Prepared client and field.			
a. Checked wound care order and specific order for irrigation solution.			
b. Premedicated the client for pain.			
c. Performed hand hygiene, donned protective eyewear and gown.			
d. Placed underpad and/or clean basin to catch irrigating fluid.			
e. Decided whether the procedure should be clean or sterile. Set up clean or sterile field by opening irrigation tray. Opened packages of sterile dressings.			
f. Poured solution into the sterile basin.			
2. Removed old dressing using clean gloves.			
3. Irrigated wound.			
a. Donned sterile gloves.			
b. Filled syringe with solution.			
c. With tip of needle about 2 inches above wound bed, flushed with slow continuous pressure.			
d. Repeated Step 3c as needed.			
4. Applied new dressing. Performed hand hygiene.			
a. Redressed wound with wet-to-moist packing and dried outer dressing as needed.			
b. Disposed of used supplies according to standard precautions.			
5. Documented client's tolerance of wound irrigation and dressing change. Documented description of wound bed.			

Additional Comments:

Name _____   Specific Skill Performed _____

Date _____   Attempt Number _____

Instructor _____   PASS _____ FAIL _____

Performance Checklist 26–2:   Removing a Dressing

	S	U	Comments
1. Performed hand hygiene and applied gloves.			
2. Removed dressing.			
a. Gently removed old dressing by pulling tape toward dressing and parallel to skin.			
b. Simultaneously applied pressure to client's skin at edge of tape to prevent skin from being pulled with tape.			
3. Observed removed dressing for drainage, especially noting amount, color, and odor (if any) of drainage.			
4. Disposed of dressing according to facility policy and government regulations. Removed gloves and performed hand hygiene.			
5. Documented odor, color, amount, and consistency of drainage. Described appearance of wound.			

Additional Comments:

Copyright © 2004, Elsevier Science (USA). All Rights Reserved.

Name _____   Specific Skill Performed _____

Date _____   Attempt Number _____

Instructor _____   PASS _____ FAIL _____

Performance Checklist 26–3: Dressing a Simple Wound

	S	U	Comments
1. Answered client's questions about procedure.			
2. Confirmed dressing order.			
3. Assembled supplies needed for dressing application.			
4. Performed hand hygiene and applied gloves.			
5. Removed dressing from its package and applied it to center of wound.			
6. Secured edges of dressing to client's skin with tape.			
7. Stated that if dressing will be changed frequently or if client has sensitive or impaired skin, to consider using Montgomery straps rather than tape.			
8. Removed gloves and performed hand hygiene.			

Additional Comments:

Copyright © 2004, Elsevier Science (USA). All Rights Reserved.

Name _____   Specific Skill Performed _____

Date _____   Attempt Number _____

Instructor _____   PASS _____ FAIL _____

Performance Checklist 26–4:   Culturing a Wound

	S	U	Comments
1. Performed hand hygiene and applied gloves.			
2. Rinsed or irrigated wound thoroughly with sterile normal saline before obtaining culture.			
3. Swabbed entire wound bed using a zig-zag technique, starting at top of wound and proceeding to bottom of wound.			
4. Handled specimen appropriately, removed gloves, and performed hand hygiene.			
a. Placed swab in culture tube.			
b. Labeled specimen correctly and placed it in biohazard container with requisition.			
c. Sent specimen to laboratory.			

Additional Comments:

Copyright © 2004, Elsevier Science (USA). All Rights Reserved.

Name _____ Specific Skill Performed _____

Date _____ Attempt Number _____

Instructor _____ PASS _____ FAIL _____

Performance Checklist 26–5: Applying a Wet-to-Moist Dressing

	S	U	Comments
1. Confirmed physician's order and assembled needed supplies.			
2. Opened sterile dressing supplies. Used sterile normal saline solution (or another ordered solution) to dampen dressing.			
3. Prepared wet dressing.			
a. Donned sterile gloves.			
b. Twisted dressing so it remained wet, but not dripping.			
c. Opened dressing fully and fluffed it open.			
4. Packed wound.			
a. Gently placed dressing into wound.			
b. Did not pack wound tightly.			
5. Completed dressing.			
a. Covered damp dressing with a dry sterile dressing.			
b. Secured it with tape or Montgomery straps, if needed.			
c. Disposed of materials and gloves and performed hand hygiene.			

Additional Comments:

Copyright © 2004, Elsevier Science (USA). All Rights Reserved.

Name _____ Specific Skill Performed _____

Date _____ Attempt Number _____

Instructor _____ PASS _____ FAIL _____

Performance Checklist 26–6: Applying a Hydrocolloid Dressing

	S	U	Comments
1. Cleaned wound by irrigating it or lightly swabbing it with gauze soaked in sterile normal saline solution.			
2. Selected a hydrocolloid dressing of an appropriate size.			
3. Applied dressing.			
a. Applied dressing from one side of wound to other side.			
b. Used hand pressure to hold dressing in place for 1 minute.			
4. Placed hypoallergenic tape around edges of dressing to secure it if needed.			
5. Stated to leave dressing in place for 5 to 7 days, but to remove and change it if it leaks or begins to peel off.			

Additional Comments:

Copyright © 2004, Elsevier Science (USA). All Rights Reserved.

Name _____ Specific Skill Performed _____

Date _____ Attempt Number _____

Instructor _____ PASS _____ FAIL _____

Performance Checklist 28–1:   Testing Feces for Occult Blood

	S	U	Comments
1. Taught client about purpose of test and had client defecate, without voiding, into collection container.			
2. Put on clean gloves, obtained small specimen using applicator and smeared thin layer in first box of Hemoccult slide while noting stool characteristics.			
3. Repeated procedure using opposite end of applicator and another area of the stool specimen.			
4. Closed slide cover and turned it over to reverse side.			
5. Opened flap on card and applied two drops of developing solution.			
6. Observed for bluish discoloration on guaiac paper 30 to 60 seconds after drop application.			
7. Disposed of slide in hazardous container, removed gloves, performed hand hygiene, and completed documentation.			

Additional Comments:

Copyright © 2004, Elsevier Science (USA). All Rights Reserved.

Name _____   Specific Skill Performed _____

Date _____   Attempt Number _____

Instructor _____   PASS _____ FAIL _____

Performance Checklist 28–2: Preparing and Administering a Large-Volume Enema

	S	U	Comments
1. Gathered equipment and positioned client on left side with bedpan in place if client was unable to retain enema. Draped client to expose only buttocks.			
2. Checked that temperature of enema solution was warm (40.5° C or 105° F).			
3. Applied clean gloves, lubricated tip of enema tube, inserted it 2 to 3 inches into rectum.			
4. Held bag 18 inches above rectum, and allowed 500 to 750 mL solution to flow in slowly over 10 minutes.			
5. Encouraged client to retain enema for up to 15 minutes, then assisted client to bathroom or commode, or checked placement on bedpan for evacuation.			
6. Cleansed perineum, assisted client to position of comfort. Removed gloves and performed hand hygiene.			
7. Verbalized to consult physician if three enemas did not produce clear results, if enemas ordered until clear.			

Additional Comments:

Name _____   Specific Skill Performed _____

Date _____   Attempt Number _____

Instructor _____   PASS _____ FAIL _____

Performance Checklist 29–1:   Collecting Urine from an Indwelling (Foley) Catheter

	S	U	Comments
1. Gathered equipment and applied clean gloves.			
2. Observed for presence of urine at port site and clamped catheter distal to port for 30 minutes or until urine visible at site.			
3. Cleaned connection port with an alcohol wipe.			
4. Inserted 10 mL syringe with needle attached into port and withdrew 10 mL urine.			
5. Injected urine into sterile container using appropriate technique.			
6. Disposed of syringe in sharps container.			
7. Removed gloves and performed hand hygiene; labeled specimen with client's name, date, and time of collection; sent immediately to laboratory.			
8. Removed equipment and documented date, amount and characteristics of urine, and time sent to lab.			

Additional Comments:

Copyright © 2004, Elsevier Science (USA). All Rights Reserved.

Name _____   Specific Skill Performed _____

Date _____   Attempt Number _____

Instructor _____   PASS _____ FAIL _____

Performance Checklist 29–2:   Applying a Condom Catheter

	S	U	Comments
1. Utilized standard precautions.			
2. Positioned client on back and draped client to expose only the penis.			
3. Cleaned genitals with soap and water and dried thoroughly.			
4. Applied skin-protecting cream to penis and allowed it to dry.			
5. Wrapped adhesive spirally around shaft of penis, being careful not to apply too tightly.			
6. Placed rolled condom over glans and unrolled condom over adhesive liner and shaft of penis.			
7. Attached to collection system and taped tubing to leg.			
8. Assessed penis after applying condom to detect potential urine leakage, edema, and changes in skin color.			
9. Documented date, time of application, and assessment data.			

Additional Comments:

Copyright © 2004, Elsevier Science (USA). All Rights Reserved.

Performance Checklist 29–3:   Inserting an Indwelling Catheter

	S	U	Comments
1. Explained procedure to client, provided privacy, and performed hand hygiene.			
2. Gathered equipment and selected catheter of appropriate size and material.			
3. Positioned client.			
a. Female client positioned supine with knees flexed and separated.			
b. Male client positioned supine.			
4. Draped client for privacy, exposing only labia in females and penis in males.			
5. Established sterile field.			
a. Opened prepackaged catheter tray and placed it in convenient position.			
b. Placed bottom drape adjacent to female client's buttocks.			
c. Held drape by corner only and allowed it to fall open.			
d. Placed it under buttocks still touching only corners.			
6. Donned sterile gloves.			
7. Placed fenestrated upper drape in place.			
8. Inflated catheter balloon to test it for leaks.			
9. Cleaned area around urinary meatus.			
a. Poured antiseptic on all 3 cotton balls.			
b. For female client, spread labia with nondominant hand while holding cotton ball with forceps in dominant hand. Used first cotton ball to clean from top to bottom of right side of urinary meatus and discarded; used second to clean left side from top to bottom and discarded; used third to clean down the center directly over meatus and discarded.			
c. For male client, used at least two cotton balls, the first to clean around the glans penis and the second over the meatus. Retracted the foreskin in uncircumcised males.			
10. Lubricated and inserted catheter.			
a. Picked up catheter 1 to 2 inches from tip with sterile dominant hand and lubricated tip.			
b. In male clients, used nondominant hand to hold penis perpendicular to client's body and used fingers to gently encircle and stabilize penis. If resistance met, had client take deep breath while twisting (rotating) catheter; did not force catheter.			

Copyright © 2004, Elsevier Science (USA). All Rights Reserved.

Performance Checklist 29–3: Inserting an Indwelling Catheter—cont'd

	S	U	Comments
c. Inserted catheter until urine began to flow (2 to 3 inches in females and 6 to 8 inches in males) and then inserted 1 inch more.			
11. Inflated balloon by injecting 8 to 10 mL of water via syringe or according to manufacturer directions.			
12. Taped catheter to inner aspect of thigh.			
13. Established drainage system. a. Leg bag: attached catheter to inner thigh. b. Gravity drainage: attached bag to bed frame below level of bladder.			
14. Completed procedure. a. Blotted or rinsed excess solution from perineum. b. Made client comfortable. c. Discarded all trash. Removed gloves and performed hand hygiene.			
15. Documented date and time of catheter insertion, amount and characteristics of urine, and size of catheter and balloon.			

Additional Comments:

Copyright © 2004, Elsevier Science (USA). All Rights Reserved.

Name _____ Specific Skill Performed _____

Date _____ Attempt Number _____

Instructor _____ PASS _____ FAIL _____

Performance Checklist 30–1: Giving the Client a Bed Bath

	S	U	Comments
1. Performed preliminary activities.			
a. Checked physician's orders for activity and any special positioning needs or contraindications.			
b. Assessed client's ability to participate in bath even if on a limited scale.			
c. Evaluated client's need for teaching relative to skin care and planned to incorporate teaching into procedure.			
d. Assessed for presence of IV lines, catheters, tubes, casts, and dressing.			
e. Assessed client's ROM.			
2. Prepared the environment.			
a. Performed hand hygiene.			
b. Gathered equipment and took to bedside.			
c. Raised bed to comfortable working height, ensured privacy by closing door or curtains, and regulated temperature.			
d. Placed articles on over-bed table, within easy reach.			
e. Applied gloves appropriately.			
3. Prepared client.			
a. Assisted client to use bedpan, commode, or urinal.			
b. Placed bath blanket over client covering the top linen.			
c. Loosened top linen at foot of bed and removed from under bath blanket and placed dirty linen in laundry hamper or bag.			
d. Placed bath towel under head and removed pillow.			
e. Helped client move to side of bed nearest you. Made sure that side rail on opposite side of bed is in raised position.			
f. Removed client's gown or pajamas.			
4. Washed client's face and neck.			
a. Filled washbasin $^1/_3$ to $^1/_2$ full of warm water. Tested temperature of water with bath thermometer or with wrist.			
b. Put on clean gloves if there was a possibility of exposure to body fluids during bath.			
c. Made a mitt with washcloth.			
d. Washed and dried client's face using clear water.			

Performance Checklist 30–1: Giving the Client a Bed Bath—cont'd

		S	U	Comments
	e. Washed client's eyes with clear water.			
	f. Washed forehead, cheeks, nose, and perioral areas.			
	g. Washed postauricular area. Cleaned anterior and posterior ear with tip of washcloth.			
	h. Washed the front and back of the neck.			
	i. Removed the towel from beneath client's neck.			
5.	Washed client's arms.			
	a. Placed towel lengthwise under upper arm and axilla. Washed upper surface of arm.			
	b. Grasped client's wrist firmly and elevated arm to wash lower surface to arm.			
	c. Washed axilla.			
	d. Washed client's hands.			
6.	Washed client's chest.			
	a. Folded bath blanket down to umbilicus.			
	b. For female client, covered her chest with a towel.			
	c. Washed and dried chest.			
	d. If bath powder or cornstarch used, applied it sparingly.			
7.	Washed client's abdomen.			
	a. Exposed only areas being washed.			
	b. Used firm strokes to wash abdomen from side to side, including umbilicus.			
	c. Observed for signs of distention or visible peristalsis.			
	d. Re-covered client with bath blanket.			
8.	Washed client's legs.			
	a. Exposed one leg at a time.			
	b. Used firm distal-to-proximal strokes.			
	c. Placed client's foot in basin for a few minutes to soak. Did ROM with toes. Inspected feet and nails.			
	d. Dried feet thoroughly, especially between toes.			
	e. Repeated process with other leg.			
9.	Provided perineal care.			
	a. Changed bathwater.			
	b. Placed client in a supine position. If client is able to wash genitalia without assistance, placed basin of water, washcloth, and towel within reach and provided privacy. If client could not wash perineal area, draped area with bath blanket so that only genitalia exposed.			
	c. Washed perineal area.			

Copyright © 2004, Elsevier Science (USA). All Rights Reserved.

	S	U	Comments
10. Washed back, buttocks, and perianal area.			
a. Placed client in side-lying position.			
b. Placed towel lengthwise along client's back and buttocks.			
c. Washed, rinsed, and dried client's back and buttocks.			
d. Performed back massage with powder or lotion (this may also be done at the completion of bath).			
11. Helped client don a clean gown or pajamas.			
a. While client is still on one side, placed one arm in sleeve of gown.			
b. Turned client to back and placed other arm in sleeve.			
12. Assisted with hair care.			
13. Assisted with oral care, as explained in Providing Oral Hygiene procedure.			
14. Made bed with clean linen.			
15. Left client's environment clean and uncluttered.			
16. Documented significant observations and assessment findings.			

Additional Comments:

Copyright © 2004, Elsevier Science (USA). All Rights Reserved.

●

Name _____ Specific Skill Performed _____

Date _____ Attempt Number _____

Instructor _____ PASS _____ FAIL _____

Performance Checklist 30–2: Providing Perineal Care

	S	U	Comments
For a Female Client			
1. Prepared for procedure and applied clean gloves.			
a. Organized necessary equipment.			
b. Placed a protective pad or towel underneath client before placing on bedpan if doing perineal care in bed.			
c. Placed in comfortable position on bedpan, toilet, or commode chair, or bedpan in semi-Fowler's position if necessary.			
d. If care was given in bed, asked client to bend knees and separate legs.			
e. Draped with bath blanket.			
2. Cleaned perineum.			
a. Poured water or prescribed solution over perineum.			
b. Separated labia with one hand to expose urethral and vaginal openings.			
c. With free hand, wiped from front to back in a downward motion with either washcloth or cotton balls.			
d. Washed external labia. Turned client to a side-lying position and washed anal area.			
e. Patted dry with second towel.			
3. Made client comfortable.			
a. Removed equipment and gloves, and performed hand hygiene.			
b. Covered client and positioned for comfort.			
For a Male Client			
1. Prepared for procedure and applied clean gloves.			
a. Organized necessary equipment.			
b. Covered client with bath blanket.			
2. Cleaned perineum.			
a. If client was uncircumcised, retracted foreskin to remove smegma.			
b. Held shaft of penis firmly but gently with one hand. With other, washed at tip of penis. Used circular motion, cleaned from center to outside.			
c. Washed down shaft toward scrotum. Did not repeat washing area without changing to clean area on washcloth.			

Copyright © 2004, Elsevier Science (USA). All Rights Reserved.

265

Performance Checklist 30–2: Providing Perineal Care—cont'd

	S	U	Comments
d. After washing penis, replaced foreskin if necessary.			
e. Washed around scrotum.			
3. Made client comfortable.			
a. Removed equipment and gloves, and performed hand hygiene.			
b. Covered client and positioned for comfort.			

Additional Comments:

Copyright © 2004, Elsevier Science (USA). All Rights Reserved.

Performance Checklist 30–3:   Helping the Client with a Tub Bath or Shower

	S	U	Comments
1. Assessed client's capacity for self-care. Assessed tolerance for activity, cognitive state, and musculoskeletal function.			
2. Made sure that bathroom was prepared and that tub or shower was clean. Placed disposable mat or towel on floor by tub or shower. Adjusted room temperature so client was not chilled during bath.			
3. Put on clean gloves.			
4. Assessed client's ability to access bathroom.			
5. Kept client covered with bath blanket while preparing water.			
6. Provided privacy for client by placing "occupied" sign on door.			
7. Tested water temperature before client got into tub or shower. If used bathtub, filled it no more than $\frac{1}{2}$ full of warm water (105°F).			
8. Provided assistance for client while client entered tub or shower.			
9. Assessed whether client could safely bathe without assistance. If client could remain unattended, showed client how to use call signal and safety bars. Placed all bath supplies within easy reach.			
10. If client was left unattended, checked every 10 to 15 minutes to determine if help was needed.			
11. If client was not able to bathe independently, remained with client at all times. Assisted as needed with bathing.			
12. Washed any areas that client was unable to reach.			
13. Watched closely for signs of dizziness or weakness while client was in tub or shower.			
14. Helped client out of the tub or shower. Assisted with drying.			
15. Assisted with grooming and dressing in clean pajamas or gown. Removed gloves and performed hand hygiene.			
16. Helped client return to room.			
17. Assessed the client's tolerance for procedure.			
18. Left bathroom clean. Discarded soiled linen. Cleaned tub or shower according to agency policy.			
19. Documented client's response to activity.			

Additional Comments:

Copyright © 2004, Elsevier Science (USA). All Rights Reserved.

Performance Checklist 30–4:   Making an Occupied Bed

	S	U	Comments
1. Organized environment and positioned client to expose half of bed.			
a. Performed hand hygiene.			
b. Closed door or curtain for privacy.			
c. Folded full-size sheet to be used as draw sheet.			
d. Lowered rail on nearest side of bed.			
e. Positioned bed at comfortable working height. Moved client toward near side of bed.			
f. Loosened top linen.			
g. Removed spread, top sheet, and blanket in one movement, at same time pulling bath blanket over client. If top linens are to be reused, folded and placed in a chair.			
h. Placed any linen that was not to be reused in laundry hamper or linen bag. Avoided contact with uniform. Held at arm's length while removing from bed to linen hamper.			
i. Loosened bottom sheet on near side of bed. Had client roll to opposite side of bed. Adjusted pillow under head.			
j. Lowered bed position to flat unless client couldn't tolerate it.			
2. Made half bed from top to bottom.			
a. Fan-folded dirty bottom sheet and draw sheet, and tucked under client's back and buttocks as tightly as possible.			
b. Placed clean bottom sheet on bed. Started with bottom edge even with foot end of bed, with center fold in middle of bed. Unfolded to top and allowed extra length to hang over top.			
c. Fan-folded top layer to middle of bed.			
d. If contour sheets were used, fitted elastic edges under top and bottom corners of mattress. If regular sheets were used, made mitered corner. Tucked sheet well under mattress at head of bed.			
3. Placed draw sheet on top of bottom sheet. Folded edge was placed at top of client's shoulders.			
a. Placed center fold along center of bed.			
b. Fan-folded top layer toward client.			
c. Tucked excess under mattress along with bottom sheet.			
d. Smoothed out wrinkles as much as possible.			
e. If incontinence pad was used, fan-folded and placed on top of linens near client's back.			

	S	U	Comments
4. Made second half of bed.			
a. Helped client turn onto clean sheets. Raised side rail and moved to opposite side of bed. Lowered side rail on that side.			
b. Removed dirty linens, folded toward center or one end of bed. Held linens away from body, placed in dirty linen bag or hamper.			
c. Pulled clean linens over exposed half of bed.			
d. Tucked in bottom sheet.			
e. Tucked draw sheet, moved from middle, to top, to bottom.			
5. Put on top sheet and spread.			
a. Helped client move back to center of bed.			
b. Placed top sheet over client with seam side up. Unfolded sheet from head to toe.			
c. Had client grasp top sheet while you pulled soiled sheet or bath blanket from under clean sheet.			
d. Placed blanket and spread evenly over top sheet. Made sure that they are even on both sides.			
e. Made mitered corners at foot of bed with top sheet, blanket, and spread together.			
f. Pulled top sheet, blanket, and spread into a tent over client's toes.			
g. Cuffed spread, blanket, and top sheet at head of bed.			
6. Changed pillowcase.			
a. Grasped closed end of clean pillowcase at center point.			
b. With other hand, held open end of case.			
c. Inverted case over hand and forearm by pulling opening of case back toward closed end. Maintained grasp at closed end. Covered pillow.			
7. Placed pillow under head. Returned bed to its low position. Placed call light within client's reach.			
8. Positioned client for comfort.			
9. Performed hand hygiene and documented care.			

Additional Comments:

Copyright © 2004, Elsevier Science (USA). All Rights Reserved.

Name _____   Specific Skill Performed _____

Date _____   Attempt Number _____

Instructor _____   PASS _____ FAIL _____

Performance Checklist 30–5:   Making an Unoccupied Bed

	S	U	Comments
1. Organized environment.			
a. Performed hand hygiene.			
b. Raised bed to a comfortable working height.			
c. Lowered side rails.			
2. Removed soiled linens. Folded soiled surfaces inward and placed in hamper.			
a. Removed bedspread and blanket.			
b. When handling soiled linens, always held them away from body.			
3. Made one side of bed at a time. Then moved to other side.			
a. If bottom sheet was contour sheet, placed elastic bands under top and bottom corners of mattress. If bottom sheet was not contour sheet, unfolded it lengthwise and placed vertical crease at center of bed.			
b. Tucked side in along mattress.			
c. If client needs draw sheet, centered draw sheet on bed and unfolded toward opposite side.			
d. Moved to other side of bed. Removed linen with soiled side in. Held bundle of linen away from body and placed in linen bag or hamper.			
e. Pulled linen to side. Tucked top of sheet, bottom end of sheet, and draw sheet.			
4. Placed top sheet, blanket, and spread over bed.			
a. Left a cuff at top of spread.			
b. Mitered corners all together at foot of bed.			
5. Prepared bed for client to return.			
a. Made a toe pleat.			
b. Fan-folded linen to foot of bed to create an open bed.			
c. Changed pillowcase.			
d. Returned bed to its low position.			
e. Positioned call light.			
f. Disposed of soiled linen.			
6. Performed hand hygiene and documented care.			

	S	U	Comments
Making a Surgical Bed			
1. Made bed as an unoccupied bed.			
2. Folded bottom and top edges on near side to opposite side, making a triangle.			
3. Picked up center point of triangle and fan-folded the linen to side of bed.			
4. Left bed in high position.			
5. Changed pillowcase and left pillow at foot of bed or on a chair.			
6. Moved all objects away from bedside to leave room for stretcher.			

Additional Comments:

Copyright © 2004, Elsevier Science (USA). All Rights Reserved.

Name _____   Specific Skill Performed _____

Date _____   Attempt Number _____

Instructor _____   PASS _____ FAIL _____

Performance Checklist 30–6:   Providing Oral Hygiene

	S	U	Comments
1. Prepared for procedure.			
a. Assessed client's ability to participate in procedure.			
b. Performed hand hygiene and donned clean gloves.			
c. Positioned client in high or semi-Flower's position or in a lateral side-lying position.			
2. Placed towel under client's chin and over upper chest.			
3. Moistened toothbrush with small amount of water and applied toothpaste.			
4. Either gave toothbrush to client for brushing or brushed client's teeth.			
a. Asked client to open mouth wide and held an emesis basin under client's chin.			
b. Positioned the toothbrush at 45-degree angle to gum line.			
c. Directed bristles of toothbrush toward gum line, and brushed from gum line to crown of each tooth, making sure to clean all surfaces.			
d. Used back-and-forth strokes, cleaning biting surfaces of teeth.			
e. Gently brushed client's tongue.			
f. Had client rinse mouth with water and expectorate into emesis basin.			
5. Had client rinse with mouthwash if desired.			
6. Removed tooth-brushing equipment.			
7. Flossed client's teeth.			
8. Removed equipment and gloves, performed hand hygiene, and made client comfortable.			
For an Unconscious Client			
1. Prepared for procedure.			
a. Performed hand hygiene and donned clean gloves.			
b. Placed client in a side-lying position.			
c. Placed bulb syringe or suctioning equipment nearby for when client needs to be suctioned.			
d. Placed towel or waterproof pad under client's chin. Placed an emesis basin under chin as well.			

Copyright © 2004, Elsevier Science (USA). All Rights Reserved.

	S	U	Comments
2. Cleaned client's teeth and mouth.			
a. Used padded tongue blade to open client's mouth.			
b. Swabbed inside of mouth, tongue, and teeth with moist, padded tongue blade.			
c. Brushed client's teeth.			
d. Rinsed client's mouth using a very small amount of water that could be readily suctioned from mouth.			
e. Lubricated client's lips with petroleum jelly.			
3. Removed equipment and gloves, performed hand hygiene, and documented care.			
4. Left client dry and comfortable.			
For Dentures			
1. Prepared for procedure using standard precautions.			
2. Asked client to remove dentures. If this was not possible, placed gauze square on front of denture. Grasped front teeth between thumb and forefinger, pulled down gently until suction that held upper dentures in place was loosened. Loosened lower dentures by lifting up and out.			
3. Cleaned dentures according to client's usual routine or instructions on cleaning product.			
a. Soaked in denture cleanser. If unavailable, used warm water and gauze square or toothbrush to clean.			
b. Brushed denture with soft-bristle brush.			
c. Rinsed under warm water.			
4. Helped client replace denture.			
5. Used denture adhesive according to package directions if client desired.			
6. Cleaned work area and made client comfortable. Documented care.			

Additional Comments:

Copyright © 2004, Elsevier Science (USA). All Rights Reserved.

Name _____   Specific Skill Performed _____

Date _____   Attempt Number _____

Instructor _____   PASS _____ FAIL _____

Performance Checklist 30–7:   Shampooing the Client in Bed

	S	U	Comments
1. Prepared for procedure.			
a. Placed waterproof pads under client's head and shoulders.			
b. Removed pins, clips, or barrettes from client's hair.			
c. Placed bed in its flat position.			
d. Placed a shampoo board or inflated basin under the client's head.			
e. Draped a towel over client's shoulders.			
f. Uncovered client's upper body by folding linens down to waist level. Placed bath blanket over client's chest.			
g. Placed washcloth over client's eyes.			
h. Placed receptacle in position to catch water.			
2. Shampooed client's hair.			
a. Used water pitcher and poured water over hair until it was thoroughly wet. Ensured that water was comfortably warm.			
b. Applied small amount of shampoo. Using fingertips, gently worked it into lather over entire scalp. Worked from hairline to neckline.			
3. Rinsed hair with warm water and reapplied shampoo if needed. Repeated until hair was "squeaky clean" when hair shafts were rubbed.			
4. Applied small amount of conditioner if desired.			
5. Made turban by wrapping towel around client's head. Patted or towel-dried until hair was free of excess moisture.			
6. Changed client's gown and linens if they were wet.			
7. Dried and styled client's hair.			
8. Helped client to assume comfortable position.			
9. Removed all equipment and left environment clean.			

Additional Comments:

Copyright © 2004, Elsevier Science (USA). All Rights Reserved.

Name _____   Specific Skill Performed _____

Date _____   Attempt Number _____

Instructor _____   PASS _____ FAIL _____

Performance Checklist 30–8:   Shaving the Client

	S	U	Comments
1. Prepared for procedure and performed hand hygiene.			
a. Placed client in sitting position, either in bed or in chair.			
b. If using safety razor, applied warm, wet towel to client's face before beginning to shave.			
c. Applied thick layer of soap or shaving cream to client's face.			
2. Shaved with even strokes in direction of hair growth.			
3. Used damp washcloth to remove excess shaving cream. Inspected for areas that may have been missed. Applied after-shave lotion if desired.			
4. Cleaned area, made client comfortable, performed hand hygiene, and documented care.			

Additional Comments:

Copyright © 2004, Elsevier Science (USA). All Rights Reserved.

Name _____   Specific Skill Performed _____

Date _____   Attempt Number _____

Instructor _____   PASS _____ FAIL _____

Performance Checklist 30–9: Performing Foot and Nail Care

	S	U	Comments
1. Prepared for procedure.			
a. Performed hand hygiene. Donned gloves if necessary.			
b. Helped client to sit in chair if possible. If client could not sit in chair, elevated head of bed.			
c. Filled basin half full of warm water.			
d. Tested temperature with bath thermometer or by inserting elbow.			
e. Placed waterproof pad under basin.			
2. Placed client's foot or hand in basin. Washed with soap and allowed to soak for about 10 minutes.			
3. Rinsed foot or hand thoroughly with washcloth, removed from basin and placed on towel.			
4. Dried foot or hand thoroughly but gently, being especially careful to dry between digits.			
5. Emptied basin, refilled with warm water, and repeated with other foot or hand.			
6. While second foot or hand is soaking, provided nail care for first hand or foot.			
a. Carefully cleaned under nails with cotton-tipped applicator. Used orange stick to remove debris. Pushed cuticle back with orange stick. Was careful to avoid injury to skin under nail rim.			
b. Began with large toe or thumb, clipped nails straight across (if approved to do so). Clipped small sections at a time, starting with one edge and working across. Filed and shaped each nail with Emory board or nail file.			
c. After completing manicure or pedicure, applied lotion to client's feet or hands. Dusted powder between digits if desired.			
d. Repeated procedure with other hand or foot.			
7. Helped client to comfortable position, removed all equipment, performed hand hygiene, and documented care.			

Additional Comments:

Copyright © 2004, Elsevier Science (USA). All Rights Reserved.

Name _____   Specific Skill Performed _____

Date _____   Attempt Number _____

Instructor _____   PASS _____ FAIL _____

Performance Checklist 30–10: Assisting an Adult Client with Eating

	S	U	Comments
1. Prepared client and environment.			
a. Performed hand hygiene.			
b. Explained procedure.			
c. Assisted client with urinary or bowel elimination before feeding.			
d. Assisted client to perform hand hygiene and possibly complete oral hygiene.			
e. Placed meal on overbed table so client can view meal tray.			
f. Checked meal tray for client's name, correct diet, and completeness of dietary items.			
2. Positioned client appropriately.			
a. Assisted client to supported upright position or to chair.			
b. Placed client in lateral position if unable to sit.			
c. Sat next to client to assist with feeding.			
3. Assisted client to degree necessary.			
a. Assisted client to eat as independently as possible.			
b. Described location of foods on plate for visually impaired client.			
c. Prepared food items by removing food covers, applying condiments, and pouring liquids as needed.			
d. Asked client about preferences for order of eating foods.			
e. Monitored temperature of beverages to ensure not too hot or too cold.			
f. When assistance was necessary, fed small amounts at a time, allowing ample time for chewing and swallowing.			
h. Provided new foods at client request, or after three to four mouthfuls of one food.			
i. Did not hurry and created pleasant environment.			
4. At completion of meal, made client comfortable.			
a. Assisted client to clean mouth and hands.			
b. Positioned client for comfort and semi-upright to prevent regurgitation if needed.			
c. Removed meal tray from bedside area.			
5. Documented food and fluid intake as well as adverse symptoms (i.e., nausea, fatigue).			

Additional Comments:

Copyright © 2004, Elsevier Science (USA). All Rights Reserved.

Name _____		Specific Skill Performed _____
Date _____		Attempt Number _____
Instructor _____		PASS _____ FAIL _____

Performance Checklist 31–1: Performing Range-of-Motion Exercises

	S	U	Comments
1. Explained procedure to client and assessed client's ability to assist with exercises.			
2. Used head-to-toe approach if moving joints of the entire body through range of motion.			
3. Supported client's body part by cradling or cupping about and below joint being moved.			
4. Put joint through its complete ROM, but did not force it beyond where it would comfortably move.			
a. Neck			
b. Shoulder			
c. Elbow			
d. Wrist			
e. Hand and fingers			
f. Hip			
g. Knee			
h. Ankle			
i. Foot and toes			
5. Observed client for tolerance, including pulse rate and discomfort, if any. Did not exercise to the point of causing pain.			

Additional Comments:

Copyright © 2004, Elsevier Science (USA). All Rights Reserved.

Name _____   Specific Skill Performed _____

Date _____   Attempt Number _____

Instructor _____   PASS _____ FAIL _____

Performance Checklist 31–2: Helping the Client Get Out of Bed

	S	U	Comments
Without a Transfer Belt			
1. Placed bed in lowest position and raised head of bed.			
2. Placed chair or wheelchair at 45-degree angle to bed. Planned for client to get out of bed on client's strongest side.			
3. Used good body mechanics to help client to a full sitting position while swinging client's leg over edge of bed in a single, smooth motion. Supported client's upper body as it came to a sitting position.			
4. Supported client in a sitting position on side of bed with feet dangling.			
5. If client was able, had client place hands on nurse's shoulders or on mattress on either side of body.			
6. Placed hands under client's arms; placed knees in front of client's knees and helped client to rise to a standing position.			
7. Pivoted with the client toward chair, being careful not to dislodge equipment or lines.			
8. Used good body mechanics to lower client into chair slowly and repositioned client in proper body alignment. Made client as comfortable as possible.			
With a Transfer Belt			
1. Placed a transfer/gait belt around client's waist.			
2. Assisted client to stand.			
a. Stood in front of client, grasped transfer belt on both sides of client toward the back.			
b. Assessed whether client had strength to stand.			
c. When client was ready, helped to a standing position by rolling body and arms upward, pulling client with transfer belt.			
3. Pivoted client toward chair and lowered client slowly into it.			
4. Had client reach for arm rests, if available, while lowering into chair.			

Additional Comments:

Copyright © 2004, Elsevier Science (USA). All Rights Reserved.

Name _____   Specific Skill Performed _____

Date _____   Attempt Number _____

Instructor _____   PASS _____ FAIL _____

Performance Checklist 31–3: Transferring an Immobile Client from Bed to Wheelchair

	S	U	Comments
1. Obtained an assistant before transferring client.			
2. Placed chair parallel to bed before transferring client.			
3. Pulled bed out from wall, if necessary. One nurse got behind client's shoulders and upper body from other side of the bed.			
4. In unison and using good body mechanics, nurse and colleague lifted client's shoulders and legs.			
5. Lowered client into the chair and positioned in good body alignment using pillows and other devices as needed.			

Additional Comments:

Copyright © 2004, Elsevier Science (USA). All Rights Reserved.

Name _____   Specific Skill Performed _____

Date _____   Attempt Number _____

Instructor _____   PASS _____ FAIL _____

Performance Checklist 31–4:   Using a Mechanical Lift

	S	U	Comments
1. Obtained functioning lift and moved it into client's room.			
2. Placed bed in its lowest position and placed one- or two-piece sling under client. Made sure sling supported client's shoulders and buttocks. Had client cross arms across own chest.			
3. Securely connected sling hooks to lift. Raised lift to elevate client enough to clear bed.			
4. Moved lift until it aligned with chair, locked wheels, released pressure valve, and lowered client slowly into chair. Removed sling from lift and stored it in a corner out of traffic.			
5. Kept sling under client and positioned client into proper body alignment.			

Additional Comments:

Copyright © 2004, Elsevier Science (USA). All Rights Reserved.

Name _____ Specific Skill Performed _____

Date _____ Attempt Number _____

Instructor _____ PASS _____ FAIL _____

Performance Checklist 31–5: Supporting the Ambulating Client

	S	U	Comments
1. Applied gait belt around client's waist and helped client to a standing position.			
2. Stood beside and slightly behind client, and walked with client while holding onto back of belt.			
3. If the client had an intravenous pole, asked client to push the pole while walking.			
4. If client was weaker on one side than the other, walked on client's weak side while grasping belt.			
5. If client was especially weak or this was first time ambulating, asked another person to walk with you to support client.			
6. If client started to fall, did not try to prevent fall by supporting client's weight with own body. Rather, helped client to fall safely, without injury to client or to self.			
7. As client started to fall, moved feet so stronger leg was somewhat behind you.			
8. At same time, used transfer belt to pull client toward you, allowing client to slide against you, supported, as you eased client onto floor.			
9. Stayed with client until help arrived. Assessed client for injury before trying to move client. Had client evaluated by physician.			
10. Documented events leading up to fall, client's assessment, notification of physician and any action taken.			

Additional Comments:

Copyright © 2004, Elsevier Science (USA). All Rights Reserved.

Name _____   Specific Skill Performed _____

Date _____   Attempt Number _____

Instructor _____   PASS _____ FAIL _____

Performance Checklist 31–6:   Walking with Crutches

	S	U	Comments
1. Inspected prescribed crutch or crutches to make sure that rubber tips were in place.			
2. Reinforced importance of arm exercises, such as flexing and extending arms, body lifts, and squeezing a rubber ball.			
3. Checked that crutches were correct length.			
a. Had client stand.			
b. With crutch tip about 2 inches (5cm) in front of client and 6 inches (15 cm) to side of client's foot, checked that distance between axilla and top of crutch was at least three fingers' width or 1 or 2 inches (2.5 to 5 cm).			
4. Taught client how to balance using tripod position by placing crutches 6 inches (15 cm) in front of feet and out laterally about same distance.			
5. Checked with physician or physical therapist to determine which gait client needed: a four-point, three-point or two-point gait.			
a. For a four-point gait, had client follow this series of steps:			
(1) Moved right crutch forward about 6 inches (15 cm).			
(2) Moved left foot forward.			
(3) Moved left crutch forward.			
(4) Moved right foot forward.			
b. For a three-point gait, had client follow this series of steps:			
(1) Moved both crutches and weakest leg forward.			
(2) Moved stronger leg forward.			
c. For a two-point gait, had client follow this series of steps:			
(1) Moved left crutch and right foot forward at same time.			
(2) Moved right crutch and left foot forward at same time.			
6. Taught client how to ascend stairs.			
7. Taught client how to descend stairs.			
8. Taught client how to get in and out of chair.			

Additional Comments:

Copyright © 2004, Elsevier Science (USA). All Rights Reserved.

Name _____ Specific Skill Performed _____

Date _____ Attempt Number _____

Instructor _____ PASS _____ FAIL _____

Performance Checklist 32–1: Turning and Moving a Client in Bed

	S	U	Comments
Turning a Client Alone			
1. Lowered head of bed and knee gatch until bed was flat; raised bed to comfortable working height.			
2. Moved client to one side of bed.			
a. Slid arms under client's shoulders and back, and moved client's upper body to one side of bed.			
b. Slid arms under client's hips, and slid hips to the side.			
c. Moved client's feet and legs to side of bed.			
3. Crossed client's arms across chest and crossed legs at the ankle. Positioned a pillow or wedge at head or foot of the bed to place behind client's back after turning.			
4. Placed one hand on client's shoulder and other on client's hip, and rolled client toward self.			
5. Turned the client far enough forward to be able to release one hand, and positioned a pillow or wedge behind client's back.			
6. If necessary, went to opposite side of bed and pulled client's hips toward center of bed to make the position more stable. Checked for proper positioning.			
Turning a Client with Another Nurse			
1. Placed bed in flat position and at comfortable working height, and moved client to one side of bed.			
a. If client was on turning sheet, student and another nurse stood on opposite sides of bed and grasped top and bottom of sheet.			
b. If client was not on turning sheet, student and another nurse stood on same side of bed.			
(1) One nurse slid own arms under client's shoulders while the other slid arms under client's hips.			
(2) On the count of three, both nurses slid client to one side of bed.			
2. Prepared client to turn.			
a. Bent client's knee on the side opposite to which client is turning.			
b. Folded client's arms over chest.			
c. Positioned self on one side of bed with another nurse positioned on other side of bed.			
3. Turned the client.			
a. If client was on turning sheet, student and another nurse stood on opposite sides of bed so each could grasp top and bottom of sheet.			

Copyright © 2004, Elsevier Science (USA). All Rights Reserved.

		S	U	Comments
b.	If client was not on a turning sheet, nurse positioned on side of bed toward which client is turning placed one hand on client's shoulder and one hand on client's hip and pulled shoulders and hip toward self.			
c.	At same time, nurse on opposite side of bed slid hands under client's bottom hip, pulled hip toward self, and placed a pillow at client's back.			
4.	Placed a pillow between client's legs.			
5.	Made sure that client was properly positioned.			
6.	If client's condition demanded that student maintain anatomic alignment of spine during procedure, used three nurses.			
7.	After turning client, documented that client was turned and the position assumed.			

Moving a Client Up in Bed

		S	U	Comments
1.	Before moving client up in bed, determined whether student could do it alone or whether help was needed from another nurse. If student planned to move client alone, determined whether to stand at the side of bed or head of bed.			
a.	For one nurse to move client up in bed from side of bed:			
(1)	Had client bend knees and place feet flat on bed.			
(2)	Placed one hand under client's back and one under thighs, close to hips.			
(3)	Told client to push legs on the count of three, and slid client up toward head of bed.			
b.	For one nurse to move client from head of bed:			
(1)	Started by removing headboard from bed.			
(2)	Placed bed in a slight Trendelenburg position.			
(3)	Slid hands under client's shoulders and pulled client toward self.			
(4)	If possible, used turning sheet to perform this maneuver.			
2.	If client had good upper body strength, used trapeze to move client up in bed.			
a.	Placed a trapeze over the bed.			
b.	Had the client bend knees and place feet flat on bed to push.			
c.	Had client hold onto trapeze and pull with arms to lift hips slightly off bed.			
d.	With hips lifted, had client push with legs.			
e.	Assisted by placing hands under client's thighs, close to hips.			
3.	If client was too heavy, solicited help from a colleague.			
a.	Stood on opposite sides of client's bed.			

Copyright © 2004, Elsevier Science (USA). All Rights Reserved.

	S	U	Comments
b. Had client bend knees and place feet flat on bed. Student and other nurse grasped turning sheet with one hand at level of client's shoulders and other hand at level of client's hips.			
c. On count of three, had client push with legs as student and other nurse slid torso up in bed.			
4. After moving client up, raised head of bed and checked position of bed.			
5. Documented that client was repositioned and position assumed.			
Moving a Client from a Bed to a Stretcher			
1. Determined need to move client (client unable).			
a. Ensured that two caregivers were positioned on each side of stretcher.			
b. Designated one person to ensure that client's head was protected during move, while other ensured feet were protected.			
c. Locked wheels on both bed and stretcher.			
d. Positioned bed and stretcher next to each other without any gaps between.			
2. Used a sheet to make transfer easier.			
a. Untucked sheet from client's bed.			
b. Grasped sheet under client's shoulders while another nurse on same side grasped it at client's hips and legs.			
c. On a count of three, all slid client onto stretcher.			
3. As an alternative, used transfer board.			
a. Student and another nurse standing on same side of bed turned client away from stretcher.			
b. Placed transfer board where client was lying and turned client back onto board.			
c. Pulled board onto stretcher with client on it.			
d. Turned client again to remove board.			
4. Raised side rails on outside of stretcher, then moved between bed and stretcher and raised remaining side rails.			
5. If stretcher could not be positioned adjacent to bed, used a three-person lift to transfer client with three nurses on same side of bed.			
a. Slid hands and arms under client's head and shoulders. Another nurse slid hands under client's back and buttocks, and third nurse slid hands under legs and thighs.			
b. On count of three, nurses simultaneously lifted client.			
c. Walked as a unit to rotate and carry client to stretcher.			
6. Ensured client comfort and safety.			
a. Covered client with a sheet.			

Copyright © 2004, Elsevier Science (USA). All Rights Reserved.

		S	U	Comments
b.	Supplied client with a pillow and raised head of stretcher if needed.			
c.	Fastened a safety strap over client.			
d.	Put side rails up.			

Additional Comments:

Copyright © 2004, Elsevier Science (USA). All Rights Reserved.

Name _____   Specific Skill Performed _____

Date _____   Attempt Number _____

Instructor _____   PASS _____ FAIL _____

Performance Checklist 32–2:   Applying Antiembolism Stockings

	S	U	Comments
1. Checked physician's order and placed client supine in bed with legs horizontal for 15 minutes before first application.			
2. Measured client's legs to determine correct stocking size.			
a. For calf-length stockings, measured calf circumference and distance from heel to knee.			
b. For thigh-length stockings, measured calf and thigh circumference and distance from heel to thigh.			
3. Placed stocking on client's foot.			
a. Inserted one hand into top of stocking and slid it down as far as heel pocket.			
b. Grasped center of heel pocket and turned stocking inside out down to heel area.			
c. Carefully slid stocking onto foot and ankle, making sure that client's heel was centered in heel pocket.			
4. Pulled body of stocking firmly up client's ankle and calf, ensuring that no wrinkles formed.			
5. Checked client's toes for pressure.			
6. Repeated with other leg.			
7. Assessed client to make sure stockings were functioning properly (no wrinkles and not slid down).			
8. Stated to remove stockings at bath times and before bed to provide skin care and perform skin and neurovascular assessment.			
9. Documented size and length of stockings, time applied, condition of client's skin, any client complaints, and times stockings were removed and reapplied.			

Additional Comments:

Copyright © 2004, Elsevier Science (USA). All Rights Reserved.

Name _____   Specific Skill Performed _____

Date _____   Attempt Number _____

Instructor _____   PASS _____ FAIL _____

Performance Checklist 32–3:   Using a Sequential Compression Device

	S	U	Comments
1. Checked physician's order and placed client in a supine position with legs horizontal.			
2. Applied antiembolism stockings.			
3. Measured circumference of client's upper thigh.			
4. Opened inflatable sleeve on the flat bed, cotton side up, and placed client's leg on sleeve.			
5. Wrapped sleeve snugly around client's leg, beginning with side that did not contain tubes. Fastened sleeve with Velcro fasteners.			
6. Connected tubing on the sleeve to the compression controller.			
7. Followed physician's orders in setting controller to correct amount and time of compression. After turning it on, observed to make sure unit was working.			
8. Documented date and time sleeves were applied and assessment findings.			

Additional Comments:

Copyright © 2004, Elsevier Science (USA). All Rights Reserved.

Name _____ Specific Skill Performed _____

Date _____ Attempt Number _____

Instructor _____ PASS _____ FAIL _____

Performance Checklist 33–1: Endotracheal Suctioning

	S	U	Comments
1. Identified need for suctioning (wet gurgling respirations with nonproductive cough or bubbling rhonchi in nasotracheal or endotracheal tube).			
2. Gathered the equipment.			
3. Determined whether to use sterile or clean technique (sterile in acute care, clean in home setting).			
4. Explained procedure to client.			
5. Set up equipment.			
a. Turned on suction (80-120 mm Hg adult, 80-115 mm Hg child, 60-100 mm Hg infant).			
b. Opened sterile saline bottle and place cap inverted on clean surface.			
c. Opened suction kit.			
d. Carefully picked up plastic or cardboard container to hold saline, squeezed to open, and set aside.			
e. Poured solution into container.			
f. Donned sterile gloves.			
g. Picked up sterile catheter with dominant hand and unsterile suction tubing with nondominant hand.			
h. Connected catheter to tubing, keeping dominant hand and suction catheter sterile.			
i. Test the suction with sterile saline.			
6. Hyperoxygenated client and correctly instructed partner in hyperoxygenation (deep breaths of manual ventilation bag as appropriate).			
7. Passed catheter and suctioned.			
a. Inserted suction catheter via nasopharynx, endotracheal tube or tracheostomy tube.			
b. Refrained from applying suction during catheter insertion.			
c. Applied intermittent suction on removing catheter; limited suction time to 10 seconds.			
8. Hyperoxygenated client again and assessed results; repeated procedure if needed; suctioned maximum of 3 passes.			
9. Used standard precautions in disposing of equipment.			
10. Documented procedure and results.			

Additional Comments:

Copyright © 2004, Elsevier Science (USA). All Rights Reserved.

Name _____   Specific Skill Performed _____

Date _____   Attempt Number _____

Instructor _____   PASS _____ FAIL _____

Performance Checklist 33–2: Administering Oxygen

	S	U	Comments
1. Assessed need for oxygen and verified physician order.			
2. Gathered equipment.			
3. Explained rationale for oxygen order and procedure to client.			
4. Set up system.			
a. Inserted flowmeter into oxygen source.			
b. Attached connecting tube and oxygen delivery device; added extra tubing if needed.			
c. Check function of system after establishing oxygen flow.			
d. Observed for bubbling in water used for humidification.			
5. Correctly applied oxygen delivery device on client and made client comfortable.			
a. Adjusted strap comfortably around client's head.			
b. Prevented pressure behind ears.			
c. Stated to use water-soluble lubricant if needed to relieve irritation to external nares.			
6. Reassessed client and system (signs and symptoms of oxygen deficit, liter flow, humidity, position of device).			
7. Documented procedure and assessment data.			

Additional Comments:

Copyright © 2004, Elsevier Science (USA). All Rights Reserved.

Name _____   Specific Skill Performed _____

Date _____   Attempt Number _____

Instructor _____   PASS _____ FAIL _____

Performance Checklist 33–3:   Cleaning a Tracheostomy Site

	S	U	Comments
1. Gathered equipment.			
2. Prepared client.			
a. Suctioned tracheostomy.			
b. Removed soiled dressing using standard precautions.			
3. Set up sterile field.			
a. Opened tracheostomy care tray touching outer corners of wrap. Uncapped bottles of solution and placed caps inverted on clean surface.			
b. Donned one sterile glove and separated items on tray with that hand.			
c. Poured hydrogen peroxide and normal saline into containers with ungloved hand according to agency policy.			
d. Donned other sterile glove.			
4. Cleaned inner cannula.			
a. Unlocked and removed inner cannula.			
b. If inner cannula reusable, cleaned inside and out with peroxide and rinsed in saline; discarded if disposable inner cannula used.			
c. Replaced inner cannula and locked it into position.			
5. Cleaned tracheostomy site.			
a. Used saline to clean skin.			
b. Used hydrogen peroxide to clean external tube.			
c. Cleansed from clean area to dirty using gauze or cotton-tipped applicator, according to amount of secretions.			
6. Changed tracheostomy ties.			
a. Protected tracheostomy from accidental removal by having second person hold tracheostomy during change of ties.			
b. Ensured that ties tight enough so that one finger can be slipped under tie.			
c. Protected client from discomfort.			
7. Disposed of equipment properly. Performed hand hygiene. Documented procedure and assessment of skin and tube.			

Additional Comments:

Copyright © 2004, Elsevier Science (USA). All Rights Reserved.

Name _____   Specific Skill Performed _____

Date _____   Attempt Number _____

Instructor _____   PASS _____ FAIL _____

Performance Checklist 34–1:   Administering Blood

	S	U	Comments
1. Verbalized to check physician's order, verified that blood was ready in blood bank, and checked for allergies.			
2. Verbalized to assess client allergies or previous reactions to blood, measured vital signs, ensured appropriate consent, prepared equipment, and obtained blood from blood bank.			
3. Verified with another registered nurse that the following information was correct:			
a. Client's name and identification number on the blood bank slip matched the client's identification bracelet.			
b. Blood bank slip and the unit of blood contained the same blood type, donor number, and expiration date.			
4. Donned gloves and primed tubing.			
a. Closed clamp and attached bag of normal saline to arm of Y-tubing; opened clamp, and primed arm, filter, drip chamber, and tubing below chamber.			
b. Closed clamp and attached unit of blood to other Y-arm; opened clamp, primed second Y-arm, and reclamped.			
5. Began transfusion.			
a. Opened clamp on NS and infused 50 mL slowly; closed NS clamp.			
b. Opened clamp on blood, and regulated at keep-open rate. Verbalized to maintain this rate for 15 minutes while staying with client.			
c. Reset drip rate to rate prescribed, after verbalizing that client had stable VS and no signs of transfusion reaction. Verbalized to continue to monitor VS.			
6. Completed transfusion by flushing the line with NS, clamped tubing, and disconnecting.			
7. Completed transfusion record, stated to return designated portion of form and empty bag to blood bank. Verbalized to place designated portion of form in client record, and completed documentation (date, type, and identification number of product; time started and ended; client response).			

Additional Comments:

Copyright © 2004, Elsevier Science (USA). All Rights Reserved.

Name _____   Specific Skill Performed _____

Date _____   Attempt Number _____

Instructor _____   PASS _____ FAIL _____

Performance Checklist 34–2:   Cardiopulmonary Resuscitation

	S	U	Comments
1. Assessed client for responsiveness and called for help or activated emergency response system if unresponsive.			
2. Ensured that client had an open airway.			
a. Positioned client on his or her back on a hard flat surface with arms at sides if possible.			
b. Opened airway using head tilt-chin lift method or jaw thrust maneuver.			
c. Removed visible food or vomitus from mouth if present.			
3. Determined whether client was breathing.			
a. Looked to see if chest rose and fell.			
b. Positioned ear over client's mouth and nose. Listened for exhaled air and felt for air movement from breathing on own cheek.			
4. Began administering breaths if client not breathing.			
a. Stated to use manual resuscitation bag if available. Used thumb and index finger of hand resting on client's forehead to pinch nose closed for mouth-to-mouth or used hand resting below client's chin to hold mouth closed for mouth-to-nose.			
b. Took a deep breath and closed lips around client's mouth or nose.			
c. Gave two breaths slowly, with each lasting 1- to 2 seconds, inhaling between breaths if not using a bag-valve mask.			
d. After delivering each breath, turned head and positioned ear over client's mouth and nose to listen for exhaled air.			
5. Checked for a pulse for 5–10 seconds at the client's carotid artery.			
a. Located artery using 2–3 fingers in groove between trachea and neck muscles.			
b. If pulse felt, continued rescue breathing at 10–12 breaths per minute (one every 5–6 seconds).			
c. Began compressions if no pulse felt and client not breathing.			
6. Assumed position for chest compressions.			
a. Placed heel of one hand on lower half of sternum, just above the xiphoid process.			
b. Placed second hand over first so that hands were parallel, and raised or intertwined fingers leaving only heels of hands resting on chest.			

Copyright © 2004, Elsevier Science (USA). All Rights Reserved.

Performance Checklist 34–2: Cardiopulmonary Resuscitation—cont'd

	S	U	Comments
c. Locked elbows and kept arms straight; positioned shoulders directly over client's sternum.			
7. Administered chest compressions.			
a. Used enough force to depress chest 1–2 inches on an adult.			
b. Released pressure fully on sternum between compressions to allow chest to return to normal position.			
c. Delivered compressions at a rate of 80–100 per minute, counting "one and, two and . . . ."			
8. Began standard cycle of chest compressions and rescue breaths by administering 2 breaths after 15 compressions and reassessed client after 4 cycles of 15 compressions and 2 breaths.			
9. Coordinated efforts with a second rescuer who arrived on the scene.			
a. Opened airway after 15 compressions and began rescue breathing, giving two rescue breaths.			
b. Allowed second rescuer to deliver 15 compressions before giving 2 more breaths.			
c. Stated to interrupt CPR when emergency team arrived only for intubation and connection to 100% oxygen by bag-valve mask.			

Additional Comments:

Copyright © 2004, Elsevier Science (USA). All Rights Reserved.

Name _____ Specific Skill Performed _____

Date _____ Attempt Number _____

Instructor _____ PASS _____ FAIL _____

Performance Checklist 35–1: Back Massage

	S	U	Comments
1. Gathered equipment and prepared environment for the procedure.			
a. Adjusted light and temperature, and eliminated unnecessary noise.			
b. Gathered lotion and extra blanket, and closed room door or bedside curtain.			
2. Prepared client for procedure.			
a. Raised bed to comfortable working height and lowered side rail and helped the client into a prone or semiprone position.			
b. Exposed client's back, shoulders, upper arms and sacral area, and covered rest of body with blanket.			
3. Administered the back rub.			
a. Started with firm, circular strokes at the base of the buttocks, moving hands toward shoulders.			
b. Massaged over scapulae with firm, smooth strokes.			
c. Without removing hands from client's skin, continued to use smooth strokes to the upper back and along sides of back down to buttocks.			
d. Kneaded along side of spine from buttocks to scapulae and around nape of neck. Repeated kneading on opposite side of back.			
4. Wiped off excess lotion and assisted with rearranging gown or pajamas if needed.			
5. Lowered bed and side rails, if necessary, and made sure client did not require pain medication.			
6. Ensured that any equipment or medications needed by the client were at the bedside.			

Additional Comments:

Copyright © 2004, Elsevier Science (USA). All Rights Reserved.

Name _____ Specific Skill Performed _____

Date _____ Attempt Number _____

Instructor _____ PASS _____ FAIL _____

Performance Checklist 37–1:   Inserting a Hearing Aid

	S	U	Comments
1. Checked that the battery was operating.			
2. Inspected the hearing aid.			
3. Turned down the volume, inserted the ear mold into the ear canal, and secured the rest of the aid in place according to the design.			
4. For a behind-the-ear hearing aid, secured the battery device behind the ear.			
a. Avoided kinking the connecting tube.			
5. Slowly turned up the volume while speaking to the person in a normal tone of voice.			
a. Asked the person to tell you when the volume was comfortable.			
6. If feedback occurred, checked for a problem.			

Additional Comments:

Copyright © 2004, Elsevier Science (USA). All Rights Reserved.

Name _____   Specific Skill Performed _____

Date _____   Attempt Number _____

Instructor _____   PASS _____ FAIL _____

Performance Checklist 37–2: Ear Lavage/Irrigation

	S	U	Comments
1. Gathered the necessary equipment.			
2. Examined the ear canal with an otoscope.			
3. Explained the procedure and instructed the client to avoid any sudden movements.			
4. Checked the temperature of the solution.			
5. Selected the irrigating device.			
6. Covered the client's shoulder.			
a. Tipped the client's head to the side to be irrigated and asked the client to hold the emesis basin.			
7. Placed the tip of the irrigation device just inside the external meatus with the tip still visible.			
8. Directed the fluid toward the posterior wall of the ear canal.			
9. Irrigation was steady.			
a. Did not use more than 70 mL of solution at one time.			
10. Periodically examined the ear canal with an otoscope to determine patency and cerumen removal.			
11. Tilted the head to drain excess fluid from the ear.			
a. Dried the ear canal gently with cotton-tipped applicator.			

Additional Comments:

Copyright © 2004, Elsevier Science (USA). All Rights Reserved.

Copyright © 2004, Elsevier Science (USA). All Rights Reserved.

Copyright © 2004, Elsevier Science (USA). All Rights Reserved.

Copyright © 2004, Elsevier Science (USA). All Rights Reserved.

Copyright © 2004, Elsevier Science (USA). All Rights Reserved.

Copyright © 2004, Elsevier Science (USA). All Rights Reserved.